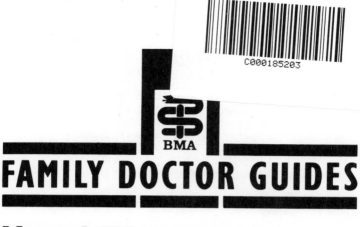

FAMILY DOCTOR GUIDES

Heart Disease

Dr Michael Petch

Series editor: Dr Tony Smith

Dr Petch is consultant cardiologist at Papworth and Addenbrooke's Hospitals, Cambridge.

Published by Equation in association with the British Medical Association

First published 1989

British Library Cataloguing in Publication Data

Petch, Michael
  Heart disease.
  1. Man. Heart. Diseases
  I. Title II. Series
  616.1'2

  ISBN 1-85336-111-9

Picture acknowledgements

Science Photo Library: pp. 20, 22, 49, 82; British Heart Foundation: p. 17; St Bartholomew's Hospital, Department of Medical Illustration: pp. 62, 68; Geriatric Medicine: p. 38; Peter Cox: diagrams; Raymond Fishwick: cartoons.

Titles in the series:

Confusion in Old Age
Gallstones and Liver Problems
Arthritis
Asthma
Children's Health 1–5
Strokes and their Prevention
Menopause
High Blood Pressure
Depression
Diabetes
Heart Disease

Equation, Wellingborough, Northamptonshire NN8 2RQ, England

Typeset by Harper Phototypesetters, Northampton
Printed and bound in Great Britain by Hartnolls Limited, Bodmin

10 9 8 7 6 5 4 3 2 1

Contents

cardiomyopathy; Restrictive cardiomyopathy;
Treating cardiomyopathy

1 Introduction

Most of us would prefer to ignore the possibility of heart disease: it can kill suddenly and without warning and it can't be cured. Moreover, coronary heart disease, which can lead to what is commonly called a heart attack, accounts for almost one out of three deaths in the western world today. This book is all about heart diseases — their cause, treatment, and the outlook for patients. Some of the facts may seem depressing, and are depressing, because I have not hidden the truth. But not everything about heart disease is doom and gloom. Advances in medicine, particularly in medical technology, have meant that most people with heart disease can now live full and practically normal lives.

Understanding is important

I have written this book for sufferers from heart disease and their families. Understanding an illness does take fear and uncertainty away and helps you to cope. I also hope that those with healthy hearts and arteries who want to keep them that way will find it useful. Although heart disease can't be cured, it can sometimes be prevented. But before we can begin to discuss the various types of heart disease, a little understanding of some basic anatomy is necessary.

Structure and function

Your heart is a muscular pump that drives the blood around your body. Blood carries the necessary oxygen and nutrients to all the tissues and organs of the body and takes away unwanted carbon dioxide and waste products. It is a dual pump. The right side of the heart receives blood from the body and pumps it through to the lungs where it picks up oxygen and gets rid of waste carbon dioxide. The left side receives oxygenated blood from the lungs and pumps it through the rest of the body.

Atria, valves, and ventricles

The receiving chambers of the heart are called atria (singular, atrium) and the thicker walled pumping chambers are called ventricles. To ensure that blood flows one way only, there are inlet valves situated between the atria and the ventricles and outlet valves between the ventricles and the large blood vessels that lead to the lungs (the pulmonary artery) and the rest of the body (the aorta).

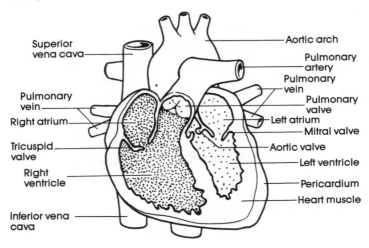

The structure of the heart.

Arteries and veins

The blood vessels that carry blood from the heart and aorta to other organs such as the kidney and brain are called arteries. They contain bright red blood that is rich in oxygen and nutrients. The blood in arteries is under high pressure. Those vessels that carry blood from other organs towards the heart are called veins. Venous blood looks blue because it is poor in oxygen. It carries carbon dioxide and other waste products and is under low pressure.

The arteries that supply blood to the heart are called coronary arteries because the early anatomists thought that they looked rather like a crown encircling the aorta at the base of the heart.

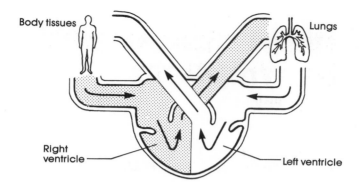

Body tissues

Lungs

Right ventricle

Left ventricle

The heart acts as a pump to circulate blood around the body. Deoxygenated (used) blood (grey) is carried back to the heart and is pumped from the right ventricle into the lungs. Here it absorbs oxygen from the air breathed in, as waste carbon dioxide is breathed out. This oxygenated blood returns to the left ventricle, from where it is pumped to all parts of the body.

How often does the heart pump?

The heart pumps regularly at a rate of about 70 beats a minute. Heart muscle contraction is called systole and the relaxation period is known as diastole. Each systole (or contraction) takes about one third of a second and pumps out about 70ml (3 oz) of blood, which means that the output of the heart is about 5 litres per minute (70×70ml) at rest. But these figures can be very variable. When you are asleep, for example, your body uses less oxygen and nutrients so your heart does not need to pump so much blood and rates of 50 beats per minute are common. But the exercising body needs more oxygen so the heart has to pump more quickly. The peak rate (roughly 200 minus your age in years) can increase output five fold in healthy people.

How is the heart rate controlled?

Your subconscious nervous system controls the rate at which your heart beats and output increases or decreases to meet the demands of the body. Electrical impulses from a group of cells in the right atrium control the contractions of the heart and these impulses travel along pathways that branch out to muscle fibres in all four chambers.

Now that we have taken a look at the structure and function of the heart we can go on to discuss the different kinds of heart disease in the next chapter.

2 Heart disease and its symptoms

Some types and terms

Coronary heart disease

There are many kinds of heart disease. By far the most common disorder, however, is the narrowing and blockage of the coronary arteries. This cuts off the blood supply to the heart muscle and causes pain, loss of pumping ability, damage to the 'electrical' system that controls the heart rhythm, and death. Various medical terms are used to describe this disease process, which can be confusing. Coronary artery disease, the term used to describe narrowing of the coronary arteries, is extremely common and often symptomless: it causes no problems until it is well advanced. Once the narrowing is sufficiently severe to reduce the blood supply to the heart muscle, however, the term coronary heart disease is used. The medical name for shortage of blood to an organ such as the heart is ischaemia, so sometimes doctors call this ischaemic heart

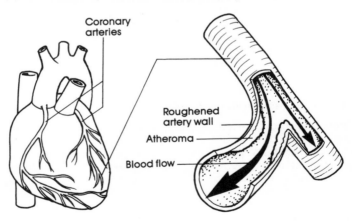

Coronary arteries can become narrowed and blocked by atheroma.

disease. Death of tissue through lack of blood is called infarction, and a coronary artery blocked by a blood clot (or thrombus) may be referred to as coronary thrombosis or myocardial (heart muscle) infarction. The popular term 'heart attack' usually means myocardial infarction or sudden death through electrical instability, both of which are usually a result of coronary artery disease.

Congenital and acquired disease

Coronary heart disease is so much more common than other forms of heart disease, that these are often overlooked. This does not matter when the overall, national frequency of heart disease is being discussed, but it does matter very much to someone who happens to suffer from one of the less common disorders. Heart disease may result from faults present at birth, in which case it is called congenital heart disease, or it may develop later on — acquired heart disease.

Features of acquired diseases

Most acquired heart disease, including coronary heart disease, is degenerative; there is a progressive structural deterioration. Degenerative diseases have a number of features in common:
- They get more common as we get older;
- Several factors are thought to speed up the process, but no single cause like a virus has been found;
- The changes in the tissues are those of wear and tear and scarring rather than inflammation.

Problem valves and cardiomyopathies

Most acquired disorders of the heart valves are degenerative. A few result from rheumatic fever, an infection which scars the valve but fortunately this is now rare in Britain. Damaged valves may be either narrowed or leaky and the medical terms for these faults are stenosis or regurgitation respectively. Hence you may come across terms like mitral valve disease, pulmonary stenosis, or aortic regurgitation. There are also some rare degenerative disorders of the heart muscle whose cause is truly unknown — these are called cardiomyopathies.

Disorders in other body systems

The heart is rarely affected by growths or tumours but it may be involved in diseases which primarily affect other organs or body systems. The most important of these is high blood pressure which imposes an extra load on the left heart. We all have blood pressure, as can be readily appreciated when the blood spurts out from a cut artery. Problems arise, however, when our blood pressure is too high, in which case damage occurs to both the left ventricle of the heart and to the walls of the arteries. The right heart may likewise be affected when the lungs are diseased and when the blood pressure in the artery that serves the lungs (pulmonary artery) is increased.

Other things that can affect your heart

The fibrous sac around the heart is called the pericardium and when this becomes inflamed or scarred the pumping ability of the heart may be damaged. Occasionally, some glandular disorders, for example, overactivity of the thyroid gland, may affect the heart. The heart may be damaged by violence, usually stab wounds or road traffic accidents. Finally the heart can be poisoned. Some drugs and heavy metals cause damage to the heart; and alcohol will weaken a previously damaged heart.

Off beat!

The sorts of structural abnormalities we have just discussed are easy to see with modern diagnostic equipment and relatively easy to understand, even though their cause is often unknown. A more difficult group of disorders, however, are those in which there is no structural abnormality but in which the rhythm of the heart is disturbed (arrhythmia). Although these disorders are extremely common, they are often short lived episodes and because of this are difficult to diagnose.

How common is heart disease?

The frequency of a disease in the population at a given time is called the *prevalence* — how many people have it now. The term *incidence* describes the frequency of a disease over a period of time, usually a year. This is the number of people who develop the disease for the first time in that year. Two other terms are important — the *morbidity rate*, the number of people with evidence of the disease, and *mortality rate*, the number of deaths caused by the disease.

Getting the sums right

There are difficulties in estimating the frequency of any disease.

Take, for example, the prevalence of congenital heart disease; that is, heart disease caused by abnormal development of the heart. If the deformity is severe, the child will be stillborn and if it is mild, the abnormality may not be detected in childhood. The prevalence of congenital heart disease depends therefore upon the age at which it is measured. In practice, the agreed definition is the number of affected children per thousand live births. The actual figure in Britain is about eight, which means that congenital heart disease is relatively uncommon.

Coronary heart disease

Similar difficulties arise in calculating the frequency of coronary heart disease, only here the problem is the long period before symptoms occur. We know that about one quarter of all deaths in this country are the result of heart disease and that coronary heart disease accounts for most of these — in 1985 there were 163 104 deaths from coronary heart disease in England and Wales. We know that in 1984, 179 000 people with coronary heart disease were admitted to hospital in England and we can calculate that in 1985, family doctors saw about 354 000 new cases. These figures from death certificates, hospitals, and GPs may be supplemented by detailed surveys of a community such as the one undertaken in Tower Hamlets, London. This survey found that each year one man in every hundred aged 45 to 64 years, had a heart attack (myocardial infarction or sudden death). In men with evidence of previous heart disease, the incidence was 12 times higher — one man per hundred per month.

A quarter of men affected

These recognised cases of coronary heart disease are only the tip of the iceberg. The British Regional Heart Survey has actually gone out to look for coronary heart disease in the community. Using a questionnaire and various techniques of examination, the survey has found that 25% of men aged 40 to 59 years show some evidence of this disease. Other surveys tell the same story; whichever way we look at the figures, coronary heart disease is extremely common and is the biggest killer in the country. Other forms of heart disease are relatively uncommon.

What are the symptoms of heart disease?

Heart disease often shows itself first as pain or tightness in the chest.

Unfortunately we all experience this from time to time and it can be very difficult to tell whether heart disease is the cause or not. Pain from the gullet, for example (a form of indigestion) can be very similar to cardiac pain. Because of this it is important to know the features of cardiac pain.

What is the pain like?

The pain of a heart attack is generally felt in the centre of the chest. It is usually severe and although it may spread anywhere, it tends to move to the jaw and arms. The pain lasts several hours, the victim feels short of breath and sick, and he usually looks awful. But the pain may be mild and not typical of a heart attack, especially in the elderly. In fact, studies have suggested that up to one third of heart attacks may not show the typical features and are not recognised at the time, only by special testing afterwards.

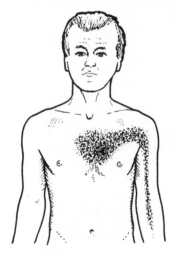

Site and spread of cardiac pain.

Anginal pain

If the arteries of the heart are narrowed, but not blocked as in a heart attack, the pain is less severe — often it is discomfort rather than pain. It comes on only when the heart is called upon to work harder such as during exercise or times of emotional stress. Usually, the discomfort builds up as a feeling of pressure in the chest as you walk and more especially if you hurry, it spreads into the neck, jaw, and arm but will subside within a few minutes with rest. This manifestation of heart disease is known as angina pectoris which literally means "strangling of the chest".

Breathlessness and tiredness

You get cardiac pain when the heart is starved of blood. But if the pumping ability of the heart is impaired, for example through valve disease or a previous heart attack, you will not have pain but instead a build up of blood in the atria and veins upstream from the heart. Since most heart disease primarily affects the left ventricle of the heart, it is the lungs that become congested and you will feel short of breath (dyspnoea). This also tends to occur on exertion and, if it is severe, it may happen when you are lying down and disturb your sleep. If your right heart is also affected, the rest of your body becomes congested and your ankles will swell. This reduced pumping ability of the heart is known as heart failure. Another symptom of heart failure is excessive tiredness, especially on effort, caused by the inadequate supply of blood and therefore oxygen to the muscles. This is, however, a rather vague complaint which most of us have some of the time, and certainly does not always mean we have heart disease!

Faints

Faints are caused by a sudden loss of blood to the brain. They may be simply due to a psychological shock, such as the sight of blood, or they may be caused by serious heart disease. The former are much more common and tend to occur in younger people. The latter occur in older people and are caused by problems such as pauses in the rhythm of the heart.

Palpitation

An awareness of your heart beat is called palpitation. This may be normal, for example after an argument or running upstairs, or it may be abnormal, for example when the heart misses beats or races for no reason (arrhythmia). The more severe arrhythmias can cause faints or feelings of faintness but usually palpitation is just uncomfortable and frightening.

The ultimate symptom

Finally, the first sign of heart disease may be when the victim drops dead. In most forms of heart disease death is usually sudden and often unexpected. The cause is a sudden breakdown of the normal, stable rhythm of the ventricles of the heart and this is called ventricular fibrillation.

3 Making a diagnosis

In this chapter we will look at the various procedures and tests available that enable your doctor to make an accurate diagnosis of heart disease.

Your medical history

Once the doctor has discussed your symptoms with you and asked a number of other questions about your current and past health he has what is called your medical history. This is always the first step in trying to establish a diagnosis of heart disease and is an extremely important part of the diagnostic process. Try to keep an open mind when you are talking to the doctor. Mistakes can be made because patients place their own (or often their wife's) interpretation upon events.

Physical examination

Your doctor will also examine you for additional clues. The things that he learns from this physical examination are called 'signs' and will include such measurements as your pulse and blood pressure. In people with coronary heart disease, however, there is rarely anything abnormal to be found.

Detecting a murmur

In contrast, people with congenital and valve disease may have no physical complaints at all. But they have murmurs in the heart which the doctor can hear by listening with a stethoscope. A heart murmur is the result of turbulence in the blood stream, similar to water rushing in a mountain stream. The murmur may be caused by an abnormal flow of blood through a defect or across a narrowed valve. Under certain conditions, however, it may be a normal finding and is simply caused by the vigorous ejection of blood in a normal heart. 'Normal' murmurs tend to be heard in slim adults and children because their heart is very close to the stethoscope and they get louder whenever the force of heart muscle contraction is increased, for example during pregnancy or when someone is anxious. Doctors can usually distinguish these so called 'innocent' or 'flow' murmurs from those that indicate heart disease.

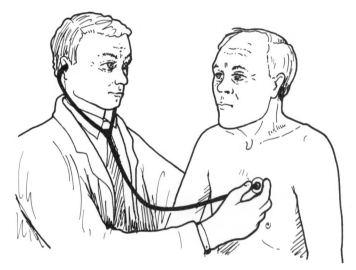

Your doctor can hear any murmur by listening through a stethoscope.

Confirmation

Often the doctor can make an accurate diagnosis from your medical history and physical examination alone. The diagnosis is then confirmed by various tests or investigations.

Tests for heart disease

Any test for heart disease can be misleading. The problems generally fall into two categories:

- False positive results, when a test gives an abnormal result and yet no disease is present.
- False negatives, when the test result is normal and yet the heart is diseased.

An especially awkward variety of the false positive test is when some abnormality such as narrowing of a coronary artery is actually present but is not sufficiently severe to affect the flow of blood to the heart and the current complaint actually arises from another organ, for example the gullet.

Interpret results with care

Tests for heart disease can thus provide false information and must be interpreted with care by a heart doctor in the context of the whole patient. If this is done, the test can provide confirmation of the diagnosis. Unfortunately, while tests can be helpful in confirming a diagnosis, they are generally less good at showing there is *no* heart disease.

Different tests

The tests available for the investigation of heart disease are set out below in increasing order of complexity.

- Electrocardiography;
- Blood tests;
- Chest *x*-ray;
- Ambulatory electrocardiography (Holter monitoring)
- Exercise testing;
- Echocardiography;
- Nuclear imaging;
- Cardiac catheterisation and angiography;
- Newer imaging techniques.

Who does the tests?

The first two tests are undertaken by most general practitioners, the next five are usually available in district hospitals, but you need to go to a specialist centre for the last two tests. The order of complexity reflects the increasing risk and discomfort to the patient, the sophistication of equipment, and the cost. The equipment cost for the first three is measured in thousands of pounds, for the next four in tens of thousands, and for the last two in hundreds of thousands.

Electrocardiography

The small electrical signals that pass through the atria and ventricles and which trigger the heart beat can be picked up by electrodes placed on the skin. The signals can then be amplified and recorded on paper. The technique is known as electrocardiography and the paper trace as an electrocardiogram or ECG. Nowadays electrocardiographic recording is very simple. Leads are placed on the arms and legs and in six positions on the chest in front of the heart. These are connected in various ways to give a 12 lead trace, which is really an electrical map of the heart.

What does an electrocardiogram tell you?

The electrocardiogram is helpful in two circumstances. Firstly, it can detect any abnormal rhythm of the heart, provided of course that the abnormal rhythm is present at the time the recording is made. Secondly, it may show the sort of abnormal pattern that occurs when there is overgrowth of the heart muscle, interruption of electrical signals, or simply loss of heart muscle. This last abnormality is found after myocardial infarction and may be fairly obvious, or rather subtle. Unfortunately, the subtle clues to the existence of heart disease may have many other causes and may occasionally be seen in normal people. It is these minor, non-specific changes that are responsible for most of the false positive diagnoses of heart disease.

An electrocardiogram is an electrical map of the heart.

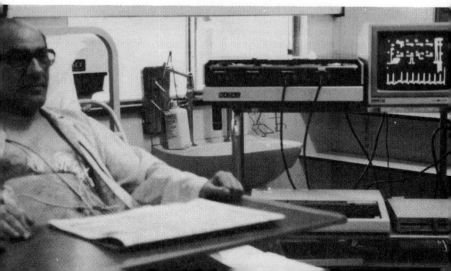

An electrocardiogram may show:
- Any abnormal rhythm (arrhythmia);
- A pattern of abnormality typical of:
  Overgrowth of heart muscle;
  Interruption of electrical pathways;
  Loss of heart muscle.

Blood tests

Blood tests are used less in diagnosing heart disease than in many other medical conditions but are valuable for two reasons:
- Measurement of the level of fats in the bloodstream may indicate whether you are likely to develop coronary heart disease;
- Myocardial infarction (heart attack) releases certain chemicals such as the enzyme creatinine kinase into the blood stream and if these substances are detected in the hours after an attack of cardiac pain a diagnosis of infarction can be confirmed.

Chest x-ray

Chest x-ray is the traditional method of obtaining an image of the heart and is still valuable in assessing overall heart size and in detecting congestion of the lungs. The picture of the heart is static; however, more detailed information about its shape and functioning may be obtained by echocardiography.

Chest x-ray should not be undertaken during pregnancy because there is a small risk that the radiation may damage the unborn baby.

Ambulatory electrocardiography

This is a development of electrocardiography devised by an American physicist called Holter. Three or four leads are attached to your chest and connected to a portable tape recorder which is usually worn on a belt around your waist. This equipment can record every heart beat for 24 hours and can be repeated if necessary. The tape is subsequently removed and played back through an analyser which can detect and automatically print out any arrhythmia.

What does it show?

Ambulatory electrocardiography is very helpful in the investigation of cardiac arrhythmias. You will be asked to keep a careful diary, so that any sensations you notice can be timed against the clock in the recorder. In about one quarter of the tests, the sensation of palpitation recorded in the diary and a printout showing arrhythmia are found to occur at the same time. In the other three quarters a less clear result is obtained partly because an apparently normal heart can exhibit a variety of rhythms which were previously thought to be abnormal, partly because the arrhythmia may be missed, and partly because people complain of palpitation when their heart is behaving normally. Nevertheless, the technique remains valuable.

Cardiac recording devices

If an arrhythmia is very infrequent, perhaps occurring once a month or less, you may be lent a cardiac recording device, either one with a memory and a capacity to store about eight 20 second recordings or one that can transmit a signal down a telephone line to an electrocardiographic recorder in a hospital. The problem with both these types of recording, however, is that the contact between the device and your skin, usually the chest or finger tips, is relatively poor and this affects the quality of the recording. Despite this drawback cardiac recording devices can complement the better established technique of ambulatory electrocardiography.

Exercise testing

Many heart conditions only cause discomfort when you exercise. People often comment that they feel a fraud when they are talking to their doctor, even though they know that with any effort such as walking to the station they are stopped by angina. Exercise testing has therefore become a routine part of the assessment of people with angina. A treadmill is usually used. You walk on a moving belt, initially at a slow speed on the flat but then at an increasing speed and slope until you are stopped either by discomfort or by the doctor who observes some abnormality. In addition to how you feel and look during the exercise your heart rate and rhythm, blood pressure and electrocardiograph will be recorded.

Sometimes a fixed bicycle is used instead of a treadmill, especially when it is necessary to keep the chest fairly still, for example when you are having some other test, such as nuclear imaging (see below) at the same time.

Echocardiography

An ultrasound beam from an electronic transducer can pass through the tissues of the chest wall and heart. Whenever the beam enters a tissue with a different density echoes are reflected back and can be picked up by the transducer and shown on a screen. Exactly the same principle is used to detect the depth of water beneath a boat. When applied to the heart, the technique is known as echocardiography. Modern echocardiographic machines can measure the chambers of the heart and this can be displayed on a moving chart so that any abnormality that occurs during the investigation can be timed. Alternatively, one part of the heart can be scanned to give a two dimensional image (2D echocardiography).

How does this investigation help?

Echocardiography can provide accurate pictures of the heart without causing you any discomfort. Satisfactory images can be obtained in most people but in some, especially those who are

Echocardiography with a single beam, narrow focus allows accurate measurement of the heart chambers.

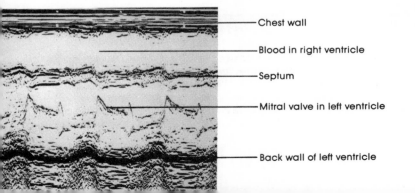

Chest wall

Blood in right ventricle

Septum

Mitral valve in left ventricle

Back wall of left ventricle

overweight, this can be difficult. The investigation is particularly valuable in identifying structural abnormalities of the heart and has greatly improved doctors' ability to investigate and understand congenital abnormalities. Nowadays echocardiographic machines can also estimate blood flow and are used to detect the severity of a ventricular septal defect or stenotic valve (see p. 63). Echocardiography signals are usually recorded on videotape and can be displayed on television screens to give truly remarkable pictures.

Not so useful for coronary heart disease

There is no better method of looking at the anatomical structure of the heart but unfortunately the coronary arteries are too small to be visualised in this way, at least in 1989.

There are also other drawbacks, including our inability to quantify some measures of cardiac function, and so other imaging techiques remain vital.

Nuclear imaging

The word nuclear has unfortunate connotations nowadays since it describes a form of warfare. Most hospitals, however, have departments of nuclear medicine which play an invaluable role in the diagnosis of heart and other disorders. The chief uses of nuclear imaging in cardiac conditions are:

- To visualise the pumping action of the ventricles;
- To estimate blood flow through the heart muscle.

What equipment is used?

The necessary equipment is a gamma camera and a supply of radioactive isotopes. A minute quantity of a radioactive substance is injected into a vein and enters your blood stream (the risks are negligible). You are then positioned under the gamma camera, which can pick up the radiation from the radioactive substance as it passes through your circulation. The data is processed later.

Cardiac catheterisation and angiography

During the past decade or so, the development of echo-cardiography and nuclear cardiology has largely replaced an investigation called cardiac catheterisation for the diagnosis of all forms of heart disease, except coronary artery disease. This is fortunate since cardiac catheterisation involves introducing a fine tube or catheter through an artery and/or vein (in the groin or elbow) into the chambers of the heart. The investigation is slightly risky, uncomfortable, can be frightening for children (and adults), and also means a stay in hospital.

How is it done?

The catheter is used to measure pressure, take blood samples, and to deliver a special dye into the heart or major blood vessels so that an angiogram, an x-ray image of the chambers of the heart and blood vessels, is obtained.

Less uncomfortable now

In the early days, the procedure was pretty unpleasant. It was accompanied by nausea and hot flushes, the x-ray film changer made a noise like a machine gun, and the patients might have to lie on a hard x-ray table for an hour or so. Nowadays, however, the images are recorded on cine film, modern dyes have few side effects, and the highly sophisticated x-ray apparatus has speeded up the investigation considerably.

Left Path of catheter in angiography.
Right Angiogram showing a total blockage in one of the coronary arteries. The blockage appears as a gap in the white artery.

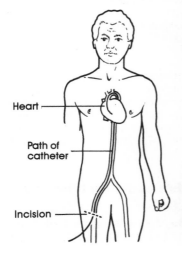
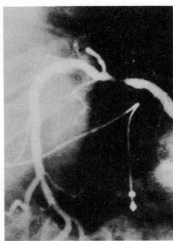

Heart

Path of catheter

Incision

Pressure and flow measurements

Cardiac catheterisation is the only way of measuring pressure in the aorta, pulmonary artery, and chambers of the heart and it is also the best method of measuring the output of blood. Because of this it is used in congenital or valvar heart disease where there is doubt about the diagnosis and when it is important to be certain, as for example before heart surgery. Accurate pressure measurements can be obtained by using fluid filled catheters connected to special pressure gauges which are attached to a sensitive chart recorder. Blood flow can be measured by several methods. In the easiest and most widely used method (thermodilution) cold salt water is injected into the right atrium and the subsequent temperature of the blood in the pulmonary artery is recorded. The cold salt water lowers the temperature of the warm blood passing through the heart and the greater the drop in temperature the smaller the amount of diluting blood and hence the slower the blood flow through the right heart.

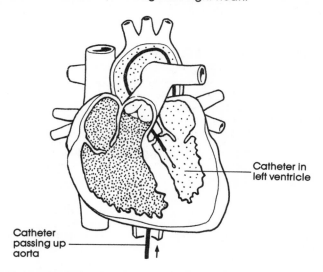

Catheter in
left ventricle

Catheter
passing up
aorta

In cardiac catheterisation a fine tube is inserted in the groin and threaded along an artery to the heart. It measures the pressure in the left ventricle and the aorta.

Looking at the coronary arteries

Nine times out of ten, the reason for undertaking cardiac catheterisation is to get an x-ray image of the coronary arteries — a coronary arteriogram. This is obtained by injecting small

23

volumes of special dye through the cardiac catheter positioned in the aorta at the entrance to the artery. Coronary arteriography is always combined with left ventricular angiography and with the measurement of pressures in the left heart. It takes about 30 minutes.

Electrode catheters

The most recent advance in cardiac catheterisation technology has been the use of electrode catheters. These special wires can be positioned in the heart so that the minute electrical signals can be recorded. Using several electrodes, the electrical pathways in the heart can be mapped, and any abnormalities can be identified. In addition, electrical stimuli can be applied to the heart and the resulting wave of activity in heart muscle can be followed. Cardiac arrhythmias can be started and stopped during this electrophysiological study, which is always done before surgical treatment of cardiac arrhythmias. These electrophysiological techniques have greatly increased our understanding of cardiac arrhythmias and remain a valuable research tool, although it must be emphasised that their value in everyday practice is limited.

Treatment as well as diagnosis

Cardiac catherisation is a diagnostic tool, but catheter techniques are increasingly being used to treat people, for example, by opening up a narrowed coronary artery with a balloon (angioplasty) described on p. 49.

Newer imaging techniques

The development of methods that allow doctors to look at the heart has been revolutionary. In particular, the use of ultrasound can now give us immediate (sometimes called real time) images of the valves and chambers so that we can see the anatomy of the heart in a way that would have been difficult to predict a few years ago. And further developments are taking place now, for example transducers are being miniaturised and can be mounted on a flexible tube which can then be half swallowed and positioned directly behind the heart to give even better images. Like many advances in the study of heart disease, this development has been made possible by improved technology; other techniques are undergoing a similar transformation.

Computed tomography

The principle of computed tomography is quite simple. Instead of a single *x*-ray beam and film, a number of film exposures are made as the apparatus rotates around the body. A computer then processes all the images so that a cut or transverse section of the body appears on the screen. Computed tomography has been invaluable in the diagnosis of internal lumps and growths and it has value in diagnosing conditions affecting the relatively static pericardium and great blood vessels. But the heart itself keeps moving and because of this clear images are not obtained. Computed tomography scanners are getting faster, however, and before long it may be possible to obtain good images of the heart.

Computer technology and angiography

Computer technology is also being applied to conventional angiography so that better images can be obtained using smaller doses of special dye. Quite good left ventricular angiograms can now be obtained from the injection of dye into an arm vein instead of cardiac catheterisation.

Advances in nuclear medicine

Advances in nuclear techniques include positron emission tomography, the use of better isotopes, and gamma cameras with greater powers of resolution. These are at the stage of improving our understanding of what goes on in the heart muscle when the blood supply is reduced but, as yet, they too have had little impact on the day to day management of heart disease.

Magnetic resonance imaging

The most exciting new technique is magnetic resonance imaging. The principle is complex but the images of the heart are good. They are not sufficiently better than those obtained by computed tomography or echocardiography to replace either of these more readily available techniques. Magnetic resonance imaging can be used to measure flow but again this is not sufficiently better than Doppler echocardiography to make it generally applicable. What does make magnetic resonance imaging unique is its ability to analyse some of the chemical processes going on in the heart muscle. At this stage it is still a research tool but it does seem to have enormous potential.

Imaging techniques for coronary heart disease

It is likely that one day one of these techniques will be able to provide images of the coronary arteries that are good enough to use in diagnosis but the machinery will probably be very complex and expensive and only available in specialist centres.

4 Coronary heart disease — causes and diagnosis

Causes

The cause of coronary heart disease is narrowing and blockage of the coronary arteries. The same process affects arteries elsewhere and blockage of the arteries to the brain will cause a stroke. The arteries of the heart are, however, especially vulnerable probably because they are continually moving — this sets up stresses in their walls which speeds up the disease process.

How do the arteries narrow?

Narrowing is caused by a gradual build up of fatty material (the lipid, cholesterol) just underneath the inner lining (endothelium) of the artery wall — this is called atheroma. The process starts early in life. The first abnormality seen is a fatty streak, and this was first noticed in young soldiers killed in action during the Korean war. The structure of atheroma in older people is more complex since it includes not only lipids (fatty material) but scar or fibrous tissue and cells from the middle, muscular layer of the arterial wall.

What happens next?

This lump (or plaque) of atheroma does not do much harm while it is covered by the inner lining of the artery but if, for any reason, a crack develops in the endothelium, events move quickly. As soon as the blood in the artery comes into contact with the atheroma, a clot of blood (thrombosis) rapidly forms. At first this clot consists mainly of sticky blood cells called platelets, but later proteins in the blood gather to form strands of material called fibrin which anchor the platelets to the wall of the artery. This clotting ability of blood is a natural defence mechanism and prevents excessive bleeding when we wound ourselves. But in the diseased coronary artery, the clot rapidly grows into the cavity, or lumen, of the artery and blocks it. Atheroma of coronary arteries may develop in small

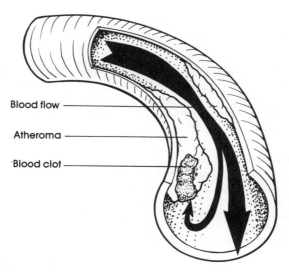

Diseased artery.

patches but it generally becomes more widespread with increasing age and in some people the whole artery may be narrowed by 'tubular' atheroma.

Muscle spasm

There is a further possible cause of narrowing of the coronary arteries and that is contraction of the muscle of the arterial wall, but the importance of this has probably been over-emphasised. Although it can certainly be seen in the arterial x-rays of some people, its importance in coronary heart disease is unclear. It seems likely that changes in the tone of the muscle layer have a small influence in angina, making it worse in the cold weather, for example. And it is quite possible that muscular contraction where there is a relatively rigid lump of atheroma could begin the process of cracking of the endothelium, which leads to clot formation. But arterial muscle spasm as a major cause of serious coronary heart disease seems improbable.

Damage does not show for some time

There is little noticeable change in blood flow through a coronary artery until the passageway is narrowed by about 80% of its original area. At that point the blood flow of someone who is resting is the same, but the narrowing prevents any increase when they take exercise. This means that the build up of atheroma has to be well advanced before angina develops (which explains the apparent suddenness with which angina appears) and even then the coronary arteries have the capacity to develop other channels (collaterals) so that when one part becomes severely narrowed, other apparently new vessels appear to bring blood from normal arteries to territory supplied by the diseased one. The development of these collateral channels explains why angina tends to disappear in about one third of patients.

No single cause

Coronary heart disease therefore does not show for some time. When angina develops, atheroma is already severe and often widespread. Cracking of the protective lining allows a clot to grow in the coronary artery and block it, causing a myocardial infarct. The essential ingredients for the development of coronary heart disease include abnormalities of the blood (of lipids and platelets) and of the arterial wall, (of endothelium and its underlying muscular layer) — there is no single cause. Instead there are a number of factors which we know to be associated with the development of coronary heart disease and these are called risk factors.

Risk factors

Risk factors for coronary heart disease are those things in life which are associated with the early development of the disease — some risk factors are powerful, others are weak. The big five are:

- Increasing age;
- Male sex;
- High blood cholesterol levels;
- Cigarette smoking;
- High blood pressure.

Many other factors have a weak, albeit fairly definite, association with coronary heart disease but usually the link is overshadowed by one of the major risk factors. For example, coronary heart disease tends to run in families. This is largely because high levels of blood cholesterol or lipid are inherited, but there is also an independent familial risk for reasons that are not fully understood.

The concept of these risk factors is challenged from time to time, and it is perfectly true that coronary heart disease can develop in some people who have no risk factors. But only five of the 202 people with serious coronary heart disease studied in the British

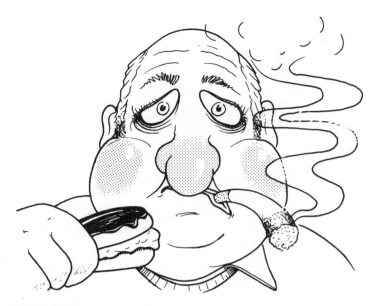

Risk factors for coronary artery disease.

Regional Heart Survey during the first four years of follow-up had no risk factors.

Multiplication rather than division

An important feature of risk factors is that they multiply together, they do not just add to each other. So to smoke and have a high cholesterol level more than doubles your risk of developing heart disease. In fact, you can calculate your risk profile simply by knowing which of the major risk factors applies to you. The risk is also graded, for example the higher your cholesterol level the greater your risk. Someone with a cholesterol level of 3.0 mmol/l is reasonably safe. If it is nearer the upper limit of normal at 6.0 mmol/l he has a much greater risk of developing coronary heart disease, although this level would still be deemed normal in some laboratories.

Age and sex

Age is the most important risk factor and 80% of the deaths from coronary heart disease occur in people aged 65 years and over. Even so this still meant that 32 447 people under that age died from the disease in 1985. Men under 65 are approximately four times

29

more likely to die from coronary heart disease than women, but in older people the risk is nearly equal between the sexes.

Blood cholesterol

After age and sex, which you can do nothing to change, the level of cholesterol in the blood is the next important risk factor. Your cholesterol level is determined by your genes but is also affected by your diet. This inheritance is bad luck for some, particularly those with both parents affected, who will develop the disease when they are quite young. But most people who are going to have coronary heart disease inherit the tendency from one parent only and do not develop the disease until their 40s or 50s.

Diet is important. There are many people who have inherited the tendency from one parent only and it is probably they who stand to gain most from a healthy diet which avoids animal fat. Ancel Keys studied coronary heart disease in different countries and showed the relationship between the amount of animal fat in the diet of a particular nation and the rate of coronary heart disease for that nation. There are, however, some interesting exceptions to this rule. Eskimos, for example, have a high fat diet yet have very little coronary heart disease. The explanation for this probably lies in the fact that they eat a great deal of fish, and fish oils are protective.

Cigarettes and high blood pressure

Smoking and high blood pressure are the other risk factors that we have influence over. The risk of developing coronary heart disease increases with the number of cigarettes smoked and with rising levels of blood pressure. In fact the risk to those who smoke 20 cigarettes per day or more is three times greater than that of the non-smoker.

Obesity

There is a link between obesity and cholesterol and heart disease. But while overweight people are more likely to get coronary heart disease, this is overshadowed by the importance of the blood cholesterol level to such an extent that thin people often get heart attacks. In so far as there is a relationship between body build and coronary heart disease, it would seem that abnormal girth is the best predictor, better than total body mass.

Stress

The risk factor that is argued about most is stress. There is a widespread belief that certain types of people are more or less likely to develop coronary heart disease. These types — A and B — were characterised by Friedman and Rossenberg in 1959. The type A personality, said to be at high risk, is ambitious, time conscious (always rushing), tends to do several things at once, and is hostile. His counterpart, type B, is relaxed, self effacing, unambitious, and content: and he is supposed not to develop coronary heart disease. The evidence for the link with personality is based on studies in California and has been corroborated by the original authors; there is even a recent paper suggesting that treatment aimed at changing a type A personality after a heart attack may reduce the risk of a subsequent attack.

Difficult to prove. The trouble is that this work has not been confirmed by other investigators and it is not only the British who cannot be grouped into either type A or B. The chief problem seems to be that there is no agreed definition of stress. Although we all think we recognise a type A personality or someone suffering from stress when we meet him (or her), the traits cannot be measured, unlike the link with cholesterol which is readily determined. And any relationship between stress and heart disease is made all the more complex by the other 'risky' habits of the type A personality — he probably smokes, eats too much unhealthy food, and is so successful in business that he doesn't have any time for exercise. It is also difficult to understand how stress can lead to coronary arterial narrowing which does tend to make doctors sceptical about the relationship. But doctors do keep open minds and while it may be difficult to understand how stress can cause atheroma, there are mechanisms which might explain why a heart attack occurs at a particular time. There are numerous stories about people who have had a heart attack after a stressful incident but this link is never likely to be proved scientifically. It follows from this that a law court would find great difficulty in awarding damages for a claim that a particular incident had caused a heart attack. Research in this area continues and the recent suggestion that 'concealed hostility' is the best identifiable personality trait that may be linked to coronary heart disease deserves to be followed up.

Exercise

The relationship between exercise and coronary heart disease is another source of confusion. Several careful studies show that people who exercise regularly are less likely to develop heart disease but we have all heard or read about the dangers of exercise. Headlines such as *Man dies of heart attack during fun run* are seen in local papers most years and squash has an undeservedly bad reputation as a killer exercise. The answer to this apparent inconsistency is that the habit of regular exercise from youth is beneficial whereas sudden, unaccustomed exercise in middle aged, overweight men who smoke can prove fatal.

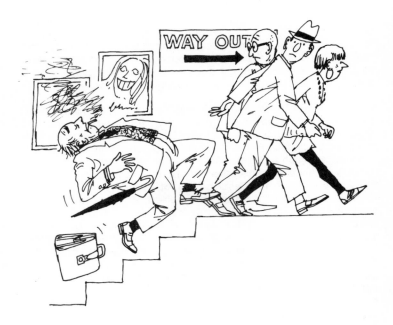

Alcohol

It has been claimed that wine helps protect against coronary heart disease. Mediterranean races, for example, suffer less coronary heart disease than we do in Britain. Their greater wine consumption is said to be part of the reason, but they do also have a much healthier diet — they cook in olive oil not lard, eat less meat, etc. The relationship between wine consumption per head of population and mortality is in fact 'J'-shaped; drink no wine and you are more likely to die of heart disease, drink too much and you are more likely to die from cirrhosis of the liver or a road traffic accident. Sadly, recent research has cast doubt on the protective effect of alcohol. The fact that those who drink no alcohol are more likely to die from coronary heart disease seems to be due to their being told by their doctors to give up because they have the disease already.

The personality and the lifestyle

So our study of risk factors helps us to identify 'coronary types' and an 'anticoronary' lifestyle. The former are middle aged men who have a family history of heart disease, smoke, eat to much animal fat, and take no exercise or alcohol. The latter are women who are born to a long lived family, survive on fish, fruit and vegetables, take regular exercise and arrange their lives to avoid any hostility. The question of whether the latter lifestyle is worthwhile is beyond the scope of this book!

National comparisons

There is noticeable variation in the prevalence of coronary heart disease throughout the world. Britain now enjoys the doubtful privilege of heading the league table. Most of the differences can be explained by the differing incidence of risk factors. Thus the high incidence in Britain is accompanied by our high cigarette consumption, fatty diet, and relatively high blood pressures. The under developed nations of the world have very little coronary heart disease. Internationally, the figures for coronary heart disease parallel those for the number of television sets in the country! This facetious observation underlines the fact that research into the cause of heart disease has uncovered associated factors, not causes.

The rates have been changing

The change in incidence of coronary heart disease in certain countries over the past 20 years is at least as interesting as the numbers at a given time. The decline in the United States has been accompanied by a similar decline in cigarette and animal fat consumption. Unfortunately no such change is detectable in Britain yet.

Rates vary within Britain

Within Britain there is more coronary heart disease in the north and west than in the south and east. The Regional Heart Survey which is based on samples from 22 towns is showing that the variation is accompanied by a similar variation in traditional risk factors. It so happens that the north and west are areas containing soft water but it now seems very doubtful whether this is an independent risk factor.

The onset of coronary heart disease

Symptoms

Chest pain is the first manifestation of coronary heart disease in about three quarters of people. As described in Chapter 1 the pain may either be that of angina pectoris or the unprovoked cardiac pain of a myocardial infarct. There is, however, an intermediate category. People sometimes come to their doctor with cardiac pain which is neither related to exercise nor typical of myocardial infarction.

Unstable angina

This condition is best called unstable angina. There are other names such as intermediate coronary syndrome, crescendo angina, pre-infarction angina, etc, but these are unsatisfactory for several reasons. Crescendo angina, for example, implies that something worse is about to happen and while this may be so, it generally is not. Unstable angina is also a useful term to describe a change in the pattern of stable angina when the pain starts occurring unpredictably. The underlying fault in the coronary arteries is probably the same as that in myocardial infarction, namely cracking of the endothelium over a plaque of atheroma, but in unstable angina the subsequent clot is partially dissolved whereas in myocardial infarction the clot grows to block the artery.

The ultimate symptom

About 10% of people with coronary heart disease will just drop dead without symptoms. This is almost always caused by the sudden onset of ventricular fibrillation — the normal rhythmic electrical activity of the ventricles breaks down and is replaced by chaotic, purposeless, electrical miniwaves so that the ventricles stop working. If immediate resuscitation is available the attack may not be fatal. We also know that only about one third of these victims go on to develop typical changes of a myocardial infarct. In the other two thirds coronary arteriography shows coronary heart disease but the ventricular fibrillation was an isolated electrical disturbance. The term 'heart attack' remains a valuable description to cover both primary ventricular fibrillation and myocardial infarction; both are serious manifestations of the same underlying disease process.

Accidental discovery

The remaining people with coronary heart disease either go to see their doctor with symptoms suggestive of heart failure such as shortness of breath or are found to have an abnormal electrocardiogram at a medical examination. The latter category is more common nowadays as routine electrocardiography becomes a part of the assessment of men in certain occupations, such as drivers of heavy goods or public service vehicles, airline pilots, and those who simply elect to undergo private health screening. Unfortunately for these men, the discovery of an abnormal electrocardiogram often leads to loss of livelihood. This phenomenon again illustrates the difficulties that patients, and indeed doctors, have in recognising the manifestations of myocardial infarction, which can be very unusual. Even experienced heart specialists have failed to make the diagnosis in themselves!

Silent heart attack

Atypical cardiac pain is more common in the elderly who may not complain of pain at all but merely feel less well than usual. But many other patients fail to consult their doctors to such an extent that surveys of populations, for example the famous study in Framingham, Massachusetts, have shown that in about one third of people who have had myocardial infarction this is unrecognised. We do not yet understand why this is so although the reasons are being studied intensively.

Chest pain is thus the first manifestation of coronary heart disease in most patients but sudden death, shortness of breath, and an abnormal electrocardiogram are also seen commonly.

Chest pain may be misleading

Chest pain is also a common manifestation of many other disorders especially those involving the gullet. But the lists of possible sources of chest pain is truly enormous and this naturally makes the diagnosis difficult. The general public is well aware of the link between chest pain, heart disease, and sudden death. Fear and worry heighten an awareness of pain so that a vicious circle develops.

Other causes of chest pain. Perhaps the most common source of chest pain is the chest wall. The chest wall is a surprisingly complex structure which comprises the back bone and its discs, the rib cage, the breastbone, and the joints between all these elements of the skeleton together with the muscles, nerves, sheaths of connective tissue, etc. Any of these can become painful and are more likely to do so with effort or emotion which increase the movement of the chest wall. Overbreathing, or hyperventilation, can perpetuate chest wall pain and bring about other sensations such as lightheadedness; hyperventilation is not an adequate diagnosis in itself, it always has a cause even if this is only anxiety.

Diagnosing angina and myocardial infarction

The diagnosis of angina can usually be established by a careful medical history. Physical examination shows no specific abnormality. The electrocardiogram of someone with angina is normal at rest but may become abnormal on exercise. The history of unstable angina is more difficult but typical cases of myocardial infarction are easier with severe, crushing, central chest pain and its attendant symptoms of nausea, fear, and a feeling of being very unwell indeed. Friends comment that the victim looks terrible. A doctor or nurse may detect the rather non-specific findings of a fast pulse rate and low blood pressure. In all these cases there may be additional clues to the presence of risk factors, for example fatty streaks around the eyes (xanthelasmata), which indicate a high cholesterol level.

In myocardial infarction the first electrocardiogram is normal in about one fifth of cases but subsequent electrocardiograms and a rise in the cardiac enzyme levels in the blood will confirm the diagnosis.

5 Coronary heart disease — prevention and treatment

Primary prevention

Prevention is better than a cure and this aphorism is only too true for coronary heart disease, which cannot be cured. Most preventive measures are common sense and self evident from a knowledge of the risk factors (Chapter 2) — don't smoke, eat a healthy diet, take regular exercise, and have your blood pressure checked. Healthy living must really start from childhood, however, and be continued throughout life if it is to be effective. The only debate in the prevention issue centres on how this advice is best put into practice.

Smoking

Smoking is associated with the development of not only coronary heart disease but also lung cancer, bronchitis, and a host of other disorders. The amount of suffering and death caused by smoking is frightening. There is no argument in favour of the habit, not even the revenue from taxation can compensate for the cost to health. Moreover stopping smoking reduces the risk of coronary heart disease after a few years. Further measures are necessary to abolish smoking in public places and to educate the young, who find the health argument irrelevant because the ill effects are delayed. Probably the best argument for them comes through pressure from employers and prospective employers; for example if two equally talented youths apply to train as aircraft pilots there is little point in training the smoker because he is more likely to have to give up his career prematurely because of coronary heart disease.

Diet

Changing the eating habits of a nation is more contentious because the gain in terms of lives saved is smaller and because there is an obvious pleasure to be sacrificed — no more pork, cream cakes, butter, chocolate . . . Since many people can handle animal fat without increasing the cholesterol level in their blood stream a policy of advising everyone to change their diet represents overkill. Yet the alternative is to try and identify those at higher risk which means that everyone must undergo blood testing in order to find out whether they are high risk individuals. Doctors are not agreed on which approach is best but the two strategies are not mutually exclusive. A reasonable policy is to encourage manufacturers to produce lean meats and label their products clearly so that people can choose what they eat; vegetable oils can be subsidised. Gradually eating habits will change. At the same time, some people, such as those with a family history of coronary heart disease, should have their cholesterol levels measured and should be given more detailed advice about diet, both for themselves and their children.

High blood pressure

High blood pressure is associated not only with an increased risk of coronary heart disease but also of stroke. It is therefore most important to identify people with high blood pressure. Measurement of blood pressure can be undertaken by general practitioners or practice nurses, nurses at the workplace, or by automatic machines at department stores. If you have sustained high blood pressure this must be treated.

What about health checks?

If screening a population for high blood pressure is worthwhile are

It is important to identify people with high blood pressure.

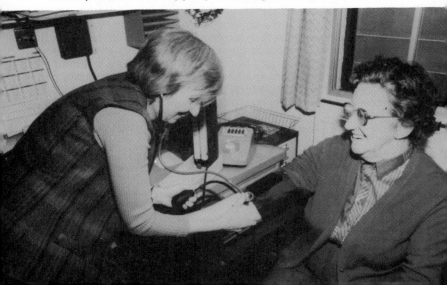

general health checks to be recommended? These are certainly available, at a price, from private health insurance companies and others. Many businesses send their executives along in the belief that good will come from the consultation but it has yet to be shown that those examinations are of great benefit to the individual, beyond the blood pressure check. Even if the routine electrocardiogram does show that the business executive had a silent myocardial infarct in the previous year, medical advice to that person would be the same, don't smoke, avoid animal fats, etc. If routine health checks were of measurable value then they would be provided by the NHS. An alternative motive for undertaking routine medical examinations, may be financial gain!

Is exercise testing useful?

Health screening centres may also offer to test your fitness. This is usually a treadmill test as described in Chapter 2. Unfortunately this cannot be recommended either, chiefly because there is an unacceptably high rate of false positive results. Many men have had to endure considerable anxiety and have had to undergo further tests, specifically coronary arteriography, only to find that their exercise electrocardiogram had been misleading. While exercise testing does help to identify those at higher risk from developing coronary heart disease, our management policy is still going to be the same — stop smoking, eat less animal fat . . .

Is screening ever justifiable?

There are a few situations where screening to identify silent coronary heart disease is justifiable. Airline pilots, professional drivers, and all those people whose sudden incapacity would place others at risk should be screened but this is best undertaken by a doctor who can handle any ensuing problems with tact and sympathy. As always, experienced judgement is better than a battery of tests.

Secondary prevention

The foregoing account is concerned with *primary prevention*, that is the prevention of coronary heart disease before it causes symptoms. Many many people will have to have their lifestyles altered in order to save a few. The term *secondary prevention* is used to describe those preventive measures that are undertaken after the disease has been discovered, for example after a heart attack. Here the measures outlined above must be applied vigorously because the benefit is greater.

Angina pectoris

The development of angina is frightening because it indicates advanced coronary disease. The medical aims are twofold:
- To relieve the discomfort so that you can continue to lead a normal life;
- To prevent a worse fate in the shape of a heart attack.

Three different groups of drugs are used to relieve angina — nitrates, beta blockers, and calcium antagonists.

Nitrates

Drugs in this group include the old fashioned but excellent glyceryl trinitrate. Like all nitrates this acts by relaxing the muscular walls of the arteries and veins. The diseased and rigid segments of the coronary arteries are probably little affected but by relaxing the blood vessels in other parts of the body glyceryl trinitrate reduces the work of the heart and thus relieves angina. The drug is often best taken just before effort since it is more effective when taken this way. The duration of action is short (some 20 to 30 minutes) and glyceryl trinitrate does not work when swallowed and therefore has to be absorbed through the mouth by sucking or chewing. The pills deteriorate in the bottle and so that a spray preparation is often better. The side effects are well recognised and equally short lived. These are headaches and faintness if you take too much of the drug or take it in a hot room with food and alcohol. Long acting nitrates such as isosorbide dinitrate are also available nowadays.

Beta blockers

The second group of drugs comprise the beta adrenoreceptor antagonists more commonly known as beta blockers. These include propranolol (Inderal, Berkolol), which has been around since 1967, and other modern equivalents such as atenolol (Tenormin) and metoprololol (Lopresor, Betaloc). These drugs act by blocking the nerve messages that stimulate the heart and circulation. They therefore reduce blood pressure and are often used for that purpose. They slow the heart rate and weaken its force of contraction so that the heart no longer has the power of a Bentley but rather that of a Mini. Because they work in this way some people become unduly tired and these drugs should definitely not be given to someone whose left ventricle is badly damaged. Beta blockers make asthma worse. Their effect on the heart is gradual and long lasting so that they need only be given once or twice a day. Beta blockers are often given with nitrates.

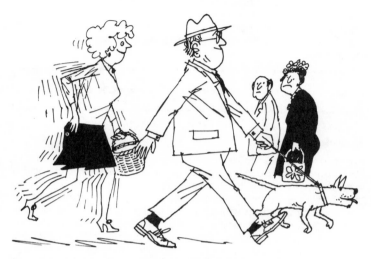

Beta blockers slow the heart rate and weaken its force so the heart works more like a Mini than a Bentley.

Calcium antagonists

The other drugs are the calcium antagonists. Like beta blockers, calcium antagonists act both on the heart and the circulation and may also be used to treat high blood pressure but the way they work is less well understood. Drugs in this group include nifedipine (Adalat), verapamil (Cordilox) and diltiazem (Tildiem). They are usually prescribed with nitrates and beta blockers but they may be used instead if there have been troublesome side effects with these other drugs.

General advice

Formerly, people with angina were given advice such as 'take things quietly for a bit'. This advice, however, had no merit beyond absolving the doctor from responsibility should a heart attack occur when the patient was doing something such as mowing the lawn. Obviously you would be ill advised to carry on doing something when your chest discomfort is present to any degree, but within that limitation you should remain active, and indeed should be encouraged to undertake physical activity. Angina will often go away with increasing fitness. You must stop smoking, you should have your cholesterol measured and a low animal fat diet should be instituted both to lower your cholesterol level and lose weight. Some people with very high cholesterol levels will need additional treatment with drugs and high blood pressure should be controlled by treatment with a beta blocker or calcium antagonist.

People with angina should be encouraged to stay active.

Hospital treatment

If the angina becomes unstable you should be admitted to hospital. At first you will be treated like someone who has had a heart attack but after the first two days or so, your progress will be much more rapid and early discharge is usual. Deciding whether angina has become unstable is a problem and will obviously depend upon circumstances. In countries like Australia where there are good resources for health care, the advice is to ring for help after 30 minutes of angina. This is what we in Britain should aim for, while recognising that it may not always be achieved.

Tests

Most patients with angina should be seen by a heart specialist and should undergo a certain amount of testing. In particular, the exercise test has predictive value since a strongly positive result often means that there may be more extensive coronary atheroma and therefore a need for coronary arteriography and perhaps more aggressive treatment. Those with a relatively negative test have a better outlook and can safely be treated with the drugs and other preventive measures mentioned.

Heart attack

Speed is essential in the treatment of a heart attack. Ventricular fibrillation means sudden death unless resuscitation is available within a few minutes. At the onset of myocardial infarction the chances of ventricular fibrillation are high and they decline rapidly thereafter. Of those victims of a heart attack who are destined to die within the next four weeks, one half do so within two hours after chest pain has started.

Coronary care units

These facts prompted doctors in the early 1960s to set aside special ward areas, known as coronary care units, to which people who had had a myocardial infarct could be rapidly transported. The doctors and nurses who staffed these units quickly became expert at identifying and correcting cardiac arrhythmias, especially ventricular fibrillation. The knowledge that most deaths occurred before the victim reached hospital prompted the development of mobile coronary care units, or coronary ambulances. These ambulances do not necessarily have to be staffed by doctors — with a little further training, ambulancemen can become adept at resuscitation and can usually get to their victim very quickly. Sadly, however, coronary ambulances are still in short supply in Britain.

Facilities for coronary resuscitation should be more widely available — in places like football stadiums, airports, railway stations — and to some extent this is being achieved. But public education in methods of resuscitation is also to be encouraged because this too can save lives.

Unclotting the blood

The second and relatively modern reason for giving people who have had a heart attack urgent medical care is so that thrombolytic treatment can be started. Attempts to dissolve (lyse) the clot (thrombus) that has blocked the coronary artery have to begin early if they are to succeed, certainly within six hours and preferably within three. This thrombolytic treatment saves lives. The drug that is used to dissolve the clot, streptokinase, has to be injected into a vein and can have harmful effects, notably bleeding. Because of this medical supervision is essential, although it is to be hoped that newer, safer thrombolytic drugs will be developed shortly.

Relieving pain

A third reason for prompt treatment is the simple, humane desire to relieve pain and anxiety. The drugs morphine and diamorphine are excellent for this purpose. Both may make the nausea that often accompanies the pain of myocardial infarction worse, however, and because of this may be given with other drugs to suppress nausea, resulting in combination drugs such as cyclimorph.

Staying at home

If you do not seek medical attention for some days after a heart attack and if circumstances permit, you can be nursed at home. Although there is no proof that rest is helpful, most doctors agree that it is desirable because we know what the heart muscle looks like after a heart attack — soft, mushy, weak and liable to give way. Commonsense suggests that effort should be avoided. Research shows that healing of the myocardial infarct into scar tissue takes six weeks or so altogether and because of this prolonged bed rest for the heart attack victim used to be recommended. But the evils of lengthy bed rest — wasted muscles, bone loss, constipation, blood clots in the leg veins — far exceed the benefits and nowadays, 24 to 48 hours' bed rest and observation are thought to be sufficient. For those admitted to hospital, discharge home after seven to ten days is usual unless there are complications. Return to sedentary work at six weeks is realistic.

Advantages of going into hospital

A further advantage of hospital admission is that any complications can be identified and treated promptly. The important ones include arrhythmias and heart failure. The former may settle over time but may require drugs such as the beta blockers. The latter will cause congestion of the lungs and shortness of breath for which 'water pills' (diuretics) are necessary.

A heart attack can be devastating

Early after a heart attack you should be given advice about the future, and the later stage of your stay in hospital is an ideal time for this. For most people a heart attack is devastating, a forceful reminder that they are mortal. Coronary care nurses become expert at helping patients come to terms with this and there are also many useful booklets on the subject. Unfortunately the hospital doctor is often too busy for very detailed conversation about your future; he concentrates on organising a number of tests, whose purpose is to gauge your future risk.

Outlook

Roughly 10% of heart attack victims will die in the year after the event, 5% in the year after that, and the death rate remains above average for several years. Patients whose hearts are more severely damaged are more likely to die. This may be very obvious to everyone in that the person never really recovers from the initial attack; he remains unwell, exhausted, short of breath with cold hands and feet and all the measurable signs that his heart is not pumping properly. Sometimes, however, the extent of the damage is obvious only to the skilled observer after special testing. This form of assessment has become known as 'risk stratification'. Dividing patients into groups according to whether they have a high or low risk of dying relies partly on simple facts such as age and the existence of previous heart damage, and partly on tests undertaken in early convalescence. This risk stratification is fallible as there are always people who defy the statistics but at least we can recognise the high and low risk groups and advise them accordingly.

Longer term

In the slightly longer term the outlook depends not only on the extent of cardiac damage but also on the presence of disease in the coronary arteries, other than the one that became blocked at the time of the heart attack. This is best judged by exercise testing. Like the patient with angina a negative test implies a good outlook, a strongly positive test implies a risk of further trouble which may take the form of angina or a further heart attack. Supervised exercise testing just before leaving hospital can give you confidence by showing you that you can walk upstairs without coming to harm, and it can also serve as a guide to how quickly you are getting better.

Rehabilitation

Formal programmes for people who have had a heart attack are not readily available in Britain, at least within the NHS. They certainly offer psychological support and are therefore to be encouraged. But these programmes have no effect on survival or any other measurable outcome after a heart attack and because of this the cost is difficult to justify when resources are scarce.

Lifestyle

Steps to improve your outlook after a heart attack starts with secondary prevention that we discussed earlier in the chapter — no smoking, a low animal fat diet, regular moderate exercise, and control of high blood pressure. Beta blocking drugs have been shown to improve survival but they are not often prescribed, because the benefit is small and many patients have to be treated to save one or two lives. Moreover people do not like taking pills especially when the side effect is that they feel less than 100% fit.

Aspirin

Aspirin is a very interesting drug. It has been known for many years that it affects the platelets in the blood, effectively making them less likely to clot. Quite recently two important studies showed that aspirin improves the outlook for people who have had an episode of unstable angina and a third study has now shown a similar benefit after a heart attack. The dose of aspirin needed is uncertain but 75 to 150mg daily is probably sufficient. The usual pain-killing dose is 300 to 600mg daily but this is more likely to cause side effects such as indigestion. The beneficial effect of aspirin is not so strong that this drug should be recommended to normal people, but certainly anyone with coronary heart disease should be taking it.

Is further treatment necessary?

Most people make a full recovery after a heart attack. Most take stock of life and change their ways. An aspirin a day keeps the next coronary at bay. Retirement is not necessary and most people should return to the job that they knew and often enjoyed. Those who experience further cardiac pain or angina and those who fall into a high risk group as judged by exercise testing etc, should be referred for coronary arteriography with a view to more aggressive treatment such as surgery or angioplasty. Very rarely should these procedures be undertaken urgently but this is occasionally necessary for the gravely ill.

Surgery

In 1967 a surgeon called Favoloro and his colleagues at the Cleveland clinic described an operation in which they used the long vein in the leg (saphenous vein) to bypass a blocked or narrowed coronary artery. The amazing success of this type of bypass surgery is now well known. The saphenous vein is removed; one end is attached to the aorta and the other to the coronary artery beyond the block. Usually the vein is cut into several lengths so that three or more bypasses are performed. The actual bypass procedure takes less than an hour but from the point of view of most patients a day becomes lost.

Is bypass surgery successful?

This coronary artery bypass grafting relieves angina in 80 to 90% of people and is very safe. Most surgical units report a mortality rate of around 1% and complications are rare, although chest wall pain and subsequent discomfort are suffered by everyone and is occasionally troublesome. A subtle change in mental function is often noticed by the patient and his family but seldom by others. This is probably related in some way to the bypass machine and usually takes the form of intellectual inertia. It improves slowly over four to six months.

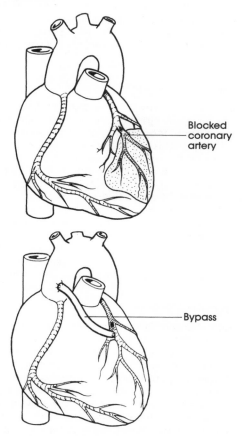

Blocked coronary artery

Bypass

Before and after coronary bypass surgery.

Internal mammary grafting

The chief problem of coronary artery bypass grafting is that the veins clog up afterwards. About 10% are blocked soon after surgery,

20% at the end of the first year, and about 50% at five years so that most people suffer a recurrence of their angina after seven years. This process can be delayed by aspirin, which should be started at the time of surgery, but even so the value of the operation is marred. Fortunately, people possess an inessential artery which runs down the inside of the chest wall near to the breastbone — the internal mammary artery. The internal mammary artery can be detached and used to bypass some coronary disease, particularly that affecting the part of the left anterior descending vessel nearest the aorta. Internal mammary grafting is not always possible but the graft does stay open longer and some 90% are still open 10 years after surgery.

Who should have this treatment?

Who then should have coronary artery bypass grafting? Clearly anyone whose angina remains troublesome despite medical treatment. But what about those high risk groups with extensive, severe coronary artery disease? Can their outlook be improved? The answer is a qualified 'yes'. We know this from two studies conducted in the 1970s, one in Europe and the other in America. Both studies recruited men with troublesome angina and compared the results of medical and surgical treatment. Both trials suggested that survival could be improved by coronary artery bypass grafting if the coronary disease was severe, affecting all three vessels or the left main stem. These findings were universally accepted because they were so obviously correct! But if the coronary disease is confined to two vessels or if the patient's angina is not troublesome, the benefits of surgery are uncertain.

It does not help in heart failure

Some patients do better after bypass surgery than others. Women are more likely to have their angina recur, probably because their arteries are smaller. Heart failure is not improved unless it is caused by a localised bulge or 'blow-out' (aneurysm) of the left ventricle which can be removed. Bypass surgery only helps when the fresh blood supply goes to active, healthy, muscle; there is no point in bringing fresh blood to dead scar tissue. Healthy muscle contains sensitive nerve endings which detect the reduced blood supply and transmit the sensation as angina; scar tissue does not. Because of this bypass surgery has value for patients with angina not those with heart failure, and very very rarely those with coronary artery disease but no angina. Some patients have difficulty in understanding why this surgery is not always recommended for them and usually conclude that doctors cannot or will not undertake the operation. The usual explanation, however, is that this surgery will be of no benefit to them.

Finally, repeat surgery is certainly possible but less successful than the first operation.

Angioplasty

The technique of coronary angioplasty is to pass a small flexible tube (catheter) with a balloon mounted on the end into the narrowed part of a coronary artery, inflate the balloon, and squash the plaque of atheroma responsible for the narrowing. The result can be quite remarkable. Your coronary arteriogram looks normal again and your angina disappears. Because the technique is undertaken through the skin (percutaneous) and because the device passes down the lumen or centre of the artery it is also known by the cumbersome term percutaneous transluminal coronary angioplasty (PTCA). The word angioplasty by itself just means remodelling of a vessel. No-one quite knows how it works but it works best in those whose atheroma is soft, which in practice means those with a shorter history of angina. One theory is that fresh atheroma is like cottage cheese and can be pushed through the outer walls of the artery by the high pressure in the balloon; another is that the whole artery is stretched at that point so that while the lumen

Angioplasty being performed. This procedure can open up arteries narrowed by atheroma.

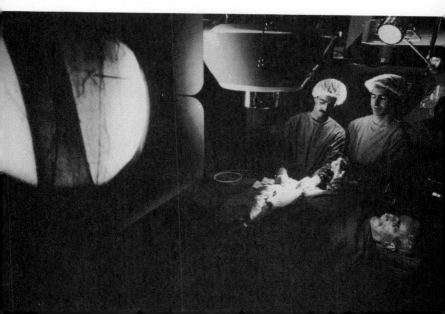

looks normal the outer wall is bulging; a third theory suggests that angioplasty only works because atheroma is eccentric, not circumferential, that is the atheroma stays put but the relatively normal arc of the vessel wall is stretched. Whatever the mechanism, it works!

Who should have angioplasty?

The technique of coronary angioplasty was first described by Gruntzig in 1977. Since then, improved materials and technology have enabled more difficult and complex lesions to be tackled. But still you will only be advised to have angioplasty if you have troublesome angina and one or two accessible narrowings. Obviously the procedure is much simpler than bypass surgery and you are home 48 hours later. The enormous drawback is that the narrowing recurs in approximately one third of patients, either suddenly through tearing of the endothelium and clot formation or gradually through accelerated formation of atheroma. Despite the use of aspirin, this complication seriously limits the usefulness of the technique. A second angioplasty carries the same success and complication rate as does the third!

6 Heart valve disorders

The most important heart valves are the aortic and mitral valves. These are the outlet and inlet valves of the left ventricle, the main pumping chamber of the heart, and are the most likely to become diseased because the stresses and strains on them are the greatest. The pulmonary and tricuspid valves of the right heart rarely become diseased, although either may be narrowed at birth, and the tricuspid valve may be damaged in drug addicts who inject (and infect) themselves.

The valves of the heart.

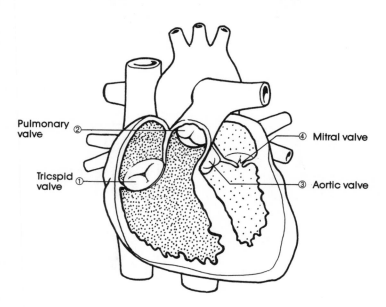

Pulmonary valve ②

Tricspid valve ①

④ Mitral valve

③ Aortic valve

Aortic stenosis and regurgitation

Stenosis of the aortic valve is a common disorder of older men in which the worn cusps of the valve become thickened and rigid with increasing age. In younger people either congenital malformation or rheumatic fever is the cause. In contrast to this thickening, the valve or its supporting tissue in the wall of the aorta

What can go wrong with the valves?

Normal opening.

Inadequate opening (stenosis).

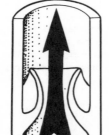
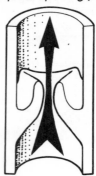

When a valve is narrowed by stenosis, the heart muscle has to work much harder to pump enough blood through it.

Normal closing.

Inadequate closing (incompetence).

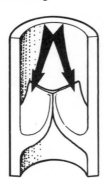
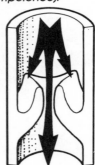

When a valve is incompetent, it allows blood to leak back into the heart. The extra work to pump it out again puts a strain on the heart.

may become thinned with age and give way so that blood leaks back (regurgitation) into the left ventricle from the aorta during diastole. This is called valve regurgitation. In either aortic stenosis or regurgitation the load on the left ventricle is increased. The heart muscle responds by beating more vigorously and by over-development (hypertrophy). Eventually, however, the heart muscle cannot cope and you begin to get angina, shortness of breath on exertion, and a tendency to faintness. At this stage, valve replacement is essential for survival because the average time between the onset of ill health caused by aortic valve disease and death is two years. Once the left ventricle begins to fail medical treatment, for example with diuretic drugs, can ease some of the problems but cannot prevent the inevitable decline. Death when it comes is usually sudden and, as is so often the case in heart disease, at a time when the victim seems to be in good health.

Mitral stenosis and regurgitation

Stenosis of the mitral valve is only seen after an attack of rheumatic fever, which is rare nowadays in Britain. A leaky valve is, however, common and is usually caused by the same sort of thinning of the valve tissue and support structures as in aortic valve disease. Part of the mitral valve may tear and give way suddenly so that you become very short of breath, but usually the 'wear and tear' is slower. Fortunately, the heart can cope with mitral valve disease relatively well and surgical treatment can be put off until your symptoms cannot easily be controlled by drug treatment. Mitral valve disease is often accompanied by an arrhythmia — atrial fibrillation — that is usually the result of distension of the left atrium. The accompanying palpitation makes you feel very uncomfortable and while the arrhythmia can be controlled by digoxin treatment, the heart rarely returns to a regular rhythm.

Mitral valve prolapse

Mitral valve prolapse (sometimes known as Barlow's syndrome) is a condition that has been discovered quite recently. Echo-cardiography has made the diagnosis easy and has established that the condition is common and affects about 2% of the population, although it rarely causes trouble. Usually it is picked up at a routine medical when the examining doctor hears an extra click or heart sound. Occasionally mitral valve prolapse causes palpitation through an arrhythmia and sometimes the prolapsing valve allows a slight leak. The cause is unknown but since it is rarely found in children, the prolapse is presumably acquired, perhaps through stretching of the thin leaflets of the mitral valve. The outlook is excellent.

Endocarditis

Any malformed valve may become infected. This infection spreads from the germs that normally live in our mouths or bowel. The resulting heart valve infection is called endocarditis. Endocarditis is serious for three reasons:

● The valve can be destroyed;

● Bits of infective material can break off and end up in vital structures such as the brain, where further damage results;

● The infection is very difficult to get rid of. Six weeks' treatment in hospital with antibiotic drugs is usual and valve replacement is often necessary.

Prevention of infection is therefore important for anyone with a malformed heart valve. This means a high standard of dental hygiene and taking antibiotics before and after having dental treatment.

Valve replacement

Heart valve surgery can be very successful in some people and as in coronary bypass surgery the operations are safe. Mortality rates for aortic valve replacement are around 1% and for mitral valve replacement around 3%. Unfortunately, however, substitute valves are not perfect. The mechanical ones take the form of a silastic ball (or a tilting disc) in a metal cage and can cause clot formation so that 'blood thinning' with an anticoagulant drug is essential. Safer drugs such as aspirin, which merely affect platelets, are not enough. Warfarin is the most widely used anticoagulant drug but to make sure that the dose is correct you have to have a blood test every six weeks or less. Despite this, there is always a small risk of bleeding. The risk of serious bleeding has been estimated at 4% per year. The alternative valve substitute is a biological or natural valve which is usually taken from a pig or

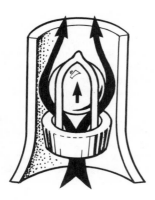 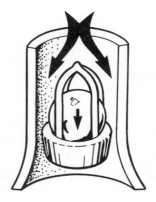

The plastic ball and cage valve. The force of blood flowing in one direction keeps the ball away from the ring, so the valve stays open. If blood tries to leak in from the other direction, the ball is forced against the ring, keeping the valve firmly closed.

Bjork-Shiley valve.

Tissue.

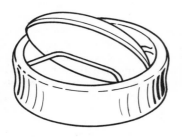 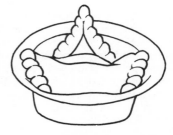

The Bjork-Shiley valve is made of metal.

The tissue valve is taken from a pig's heart.

Replacement valves.

sometimes from human donors such as victims of road traffic accidents. After careful preparation these valves can give good service for many years and anticoagulants are not needed, but they do not last forever. Although they have not been available for long enough for their life span to be determined, seven to ten years seems likely and rather less in young people.

Valve repair

The attraction of valve repair thus becomes evident. A narrowed mitral valve can be opened (mitral valvotomy) and this operation gives excellent results. A similar procedure on the aortic valve is less successful but has been undertaken in children whose hearts are too small to accommodate a replacement valve. Repair of a leaking mitral valve is gaining popularity. But all these repair procedures have limited application and whenever a patient agrees to undergo valve surgery he must accept that repair may not be possible and that he will have to end up with an old fashioned mechanical valve which, for all its faults, has proved reliable over three decades.

Valvoplasty

Just as coronary angioplasty can open up a narrowed artery so balloon valvoplasty can open up a narrowed valve. This procedure is only used for narrowed valves, however, not leaky ones. It gives temporary improvement to most of the people with narrowed aortic valves in whom it has been tried. But in children with the same problem the procedure can buy time and allow the child to develop until such time as an adult sized substitute valve can be implanted. In pulmonary valve narrowing the procedure is so successful that the balloon catheter inflation of the valve is now the treatment of choice. Early reports suggest that the procedure is likely to be successful in opening up narrowed mitral valves, as might be predicted from the success of mitral valvotomy using only the surgeon's finger 30 years ago. Valvoplasty, like angioplasty, has the great advantage that it does not require major surgery and opening the chest.

7 Heart muscle disease and pump failure

The walls of your heart are made of muscle, which can become diseased, causing a reduction in cardiac output. Heart muscle disease may be *secondary* to some disorder such as ischaemia (shortage of blood to the heart) or high blood pressure, or it may be associated with some other disease process. Alternatively it may be *primary* in which case it is called cardiomyopathy. The official definition of cardiomyopathy is heart muscle disease of unknown cause or association. There are three types:

- Hypertrophic cardiomyopathy in which there is abnormal overgrowth of heart muscle;
- Dilated cardiomyopathy in which the heart muscle wastes away and is replaced by scar tissue so that the heart enlarges (dilates) into a flabby bag;
- Restrictive cardiomyopathy where the heart muscle becomes stiff and inflexible.

Hypertrophic cardiomyopathy

In the relatively rare condition, hypertrophic cardiomyopathy, there may be so much abnormal muscular growth that the flow of blood through the heart is obstructed — the cardiomyopathy is then called hypertrophic obstructive cardiomyopathy. In either case, the muscular overgrowth is too great for the blood supply so that angina is usually the first symptom. But there are others:

- An abnormal electrocardiogram;
- Palpitation;
- Shortness of breath;
- Faintness;
- Occasionally, sudden death.

The last of these is associated with ventricular arrhythmias but these can be controlled by drugs. Hypertrophic cardiomyopathy may occur sporadically or run in families. The best diagnostic test is echocardiography. Drugs such as the beta blockers control symptoms, and surgery is sometimes helpful.

Dilated cardiomyopathy

Although the cause of dilated cardiomyopathy is unknown, that does not stop doctors speculating. We know that a very similar pattern of heart muscle wasting is seen in generalised muscle disorders, in association with other diseases, after some infections (such as one called Chagas disease), and after poisons such as heavy metals and excess alcohol. It is probable therefore that dilated cardiomyopathy is the burnt out stage of a variety of damaging processes.

Cardiomyopathy and viruses

When there is no history of such a process the possibility exists that the original cause was a virus infection which has long since passed. Certainly inflammation of heart muscle (myocarditis) can be found during some virus infections and abnormal cells, suggestive of a previous infection, can be found in heart muscle samples taken from people suffering from dilated cardiomyopathy. But the link remains unproved. Meanwhile the theory that myocarditis caused by a viral infection can progress to dilated cardiomyopathy is certainly possible. Since making your heart work too hard may accelerate the damage done by a virus infection it follows that you should not exert yourself when you are suffering from a virus infection, however trivial. Certain types of viruses, for example the Coxsackie B group, seem to be more likely to affect the heart but there is no evidence to incriminate the heart in the currently fashionable post viral syndrome, or ME.

Diagnosing dilated cardiomyopathy

Dilated cardiomyopathy may be noticed at an early stage through an abnormal electrocardiogram or chest x-ray. As the disease progresses, however, the heart muscle begins to fail and fluid accumulates in the lungs and other tissues so that you become short of breath and bloated (or congested). Because of this it is sometimes called congestive cardiomyopathy. Deterioration is slow but usually unrelenting. A very similar picture ensues after several myocardial infarcts and with the various harmful agents mentioned above.

Cause and outlook

Longstanding aortic valve disease, mitral regurgitation, high blood pressure, and all those conditions which overburden the heart for decades will ultimately lead to failure of the heart as a pump. When the heart muscle is irrevocably stretched and scarred, when the heart is flabby and enlarged, all attempts to correct the underlying abnormality, for example by valve replacement, are doomed to fail. The overburdened heart muscle will never recover. Whatever the original cause the end result is distressingly common: the sick patient with an exhausted heart and a few treatment options. In dilated cardiomyopathy the time from the *onset* of overt heart failure to *death* from ventricular fibrillation averages two years.

Restrictive cardiomyopathy

There is a third and very rare form of cardiomyopathy in which the heart is normal in size but the muscle is so stiff that the ventricles cannot fill or empty properly. This restrictive cardiomyopathy is very like dilated cardiomyopathy apart from the relatively small heart.

Treating cardiomyopathy

Cardiomyopathy cannot be prevented since we do not know the cause. Once dilated cardiomyopathy has been diagnosed physical effort should be minimised to save the heart's limited resources. Fluid tablets (diuretics) will alleviate congestion and thus ease the shortness of breath and bloated feeling and drugs are available to stimulate the heart muscle into increased activity. One of these, digoxin, is well tried but its stimulatory effect is weak. Other new drugs are being produced but as yet none has enjoyed lasting success.

Vasodilators and ACE inhibitors

Attempts to stimulate a failing heart could in theory exhaust it and thus shorten its working life. An alternative approach is to use drugs which relax the muscular tone in the walls of the arteries and veins (vasodilators). In a normal person, these drugs cause a drop in blood pressure. In someone with heart failure the drop is very short lived and the chief effect is an increase in the amount of blood flowing forward through the heart, which of course means an increased output for less work. Unfortunately, the action of most vasodilator drugs such as the nitrates is short lived and moreover, drug tolerance develops so that the drugs cease to be effective after 48 hours or so. But one group of drugs for which the pharmaceutical industry must take much credit are known as the angiotensin converting enzyme (ACE) inhibitors and these are most helpful. Captopril (Capoten) and enalapril (Innovace) are examples in widespread use. Both improve severe heart failure when given with diuretics, and may also be used in the treatment of high blood pressure. These drugs do tend to cause faintness. Enalapril has been shown to prolong life in severe heart failure.

A new heart?

The ultimate treatment for pump failure is a new heart. Unfortunately there is no really satisfactory substitute and hearts taken from brain-dead donors will always be in short supply. Mechanical devices are a temporary measure only. Retraining ordinary body muscle to function as an auxillary pump is still very experimental and at present animal hearts are unusable.

Is it worth it?

Heart transplant operations attract publicity out of all proportion to the numbers performed or their scientific importance. A few hundred heart transplants are performed in Britain each year compared with thousands of pacemaker implants, coronary angioplasties, or bypass grafts, and speaking scientifically, thrombolytic treatment for heart attacks is far more exciting. Heart transplants are also expensive. They cost three or four times more than a conventional heart operation and drugs to suppress rejection of the new heart, which must be continued indefinitely, are also expensive. A final drawback is that the operation is tinged with sadness over the death of the previously fit donor.

But results can be dramatic

Heart transplantation can produce dramatic results, however, literally saving some young people from death and restoring them to normal activity. The intense public interest is not surprising. The success rate of the procedure has improved so that 66–75% now survive the first year and some half or two thirds live for five years. The indication for surgery is usually severe dilated cardiomyopathy or end-stage coronary heart disease, and for younger people with these diseases it represents their best chance of survival. In patients over 50 to 55 years of age the complication rate is higher and the operation is not usually recommended.

8 Congenital heart disease

Congenital abnormalities of the heart are growth faults that develop before birth. They range from trivial problems that do not affect the quality or length of life to very severe defects which result in a stillbirth. The abnormalities may be classified into narrowings (stenoses) which impede the flow of blood, holes or defects which permit interchange of blood (shunting) between the left and right sides of the heart, and more complex problems.

Aortic and pulmonary stenoses

Narrowing of the pulmonary or aortic valve (called pulmonary stenosis or aortic stenosis) imposes an extra load on the pumping chamber (right or left ventricle respectively). This is generally tolerated for decades and often no further action is required. If the stenosis is severe, however, then it may be treated by balloon valvotomy (see Chapter 6). Often the aortic valve will have to be replaced in adult life but this is rarely necessary with the pulmonary valve.

Coarctation

A third narrowing is found around the arch of the aorta and this is known as coarctation. A coarctation of the aorta is shaped like an hour glass and has the effect of increasing the blood pressure in the upper part of the body. The lower part of the body then receives a reduced blood supply, largely through collateral arteries which open up in the chest wall. The condition is usually recognised at a routine medical because high blood pressure in the arms is combined with weak arterial pulse in the legs. Once diagnosed a coarctation should be treated by surgery in order to bring down the blood pressure and reduce the risk of stroke.

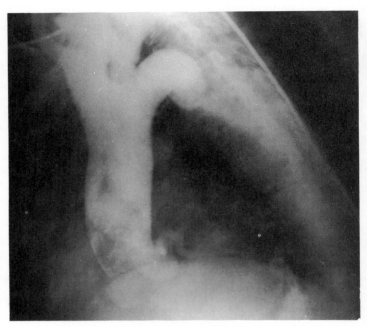

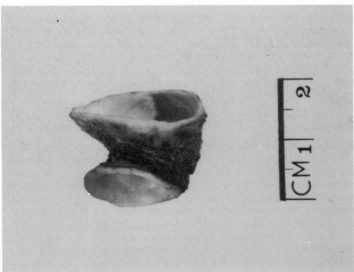

Coarctation of the aorta.

Septal defects and patent ductus arteriosus

Abnormal communications between the left and right sides of the heart may be 'holes in the heart' itself (called atrial septal defect or ventricular septal defect) or between the aorta and pulmonary artery near the site of a coarctation (known as patent ductus arteriosus). All these conditions tend to be recognised in childhood when abnormal heart sounds and murmurs are heard. In each condition blood flows from the high pressure left side to the low resistance right side thus increasing the flow of blood through the lungs. This left to right 'shunt' causes the heart, and in particular the left ventricle in the case of a ventricular septal defect, to work unduly hard. Sometimes therefore a ventricular septal defect may cause heart failure in early life. The condition is interesting in that a defect with a diameter of 0.5cm may be extremely disturbing to an infant whose heart measures 3cm but well tolerated when the heart measures 10cm. In fact some ventricular septal defects close spontaneously as the heart grows. These and small atrial septal defects may be safely left alone but any patent ductus and any septal defect that allows considerable shunting of blood should be closed.

Surgery in childhood

To recommend open heart surgery to the parents of an apparently healthy child is one of the more difficult tasks that a heart specialist has to face. Yet to do otherwise would be to condemn that child to suffer and die from heart failure in middle life. Childhood is unquestionably the best time for surgery since the heart has not had time to deteriorate from overwork, the operation does not interfere with examinations, and recovery is rapid. Surgery is very very safe, the chief problem is usually the parents' anxiety state.

Striking a balance

All the conditions described above can be confirmed by echocardiography. There is plenty of time to establish the diagnosis with certainty and discuss the child's future. Of the eight cases of congenital heart disease for every 1000 live births, approximately one third are ventricular septal defects. More complex forms of

63

congenital heart disease account for less than 10%. These relative rarities include such conditions as Fallot's tetralogy and transposition of the great arteries which generally cause trouble at, or shortly after birth. Emergency treatment may be necessary and because the chances of a normal life are slender, these conditions pose a moral dilemma. On the one hand there is the temptation to let nature take its course, especially when the congenital heart disease is accompanied by other disabling malformations. On the other hand these conditions present a challenge to medical technology and unless experimental procedures are undertaken in these children others can never benefit. In general, the right balance is struck except occasionally when the glare of publicity ensures that a child's life is preserved, sometimes at a terrible price.

Medical advances

Some medical advances in this field are a delight, for example Blalock's invention of connecting the major artery of the arm (subclavian artery) to the pulmonary artery. This operation brought blood to the lungs of children suffering from Fallot's tetralogy in which the combination of pulmonary stenosis and a ventricular septal defect had previously resulted in most blood going from the right ventricle to the aorta, thus avoiding the lungs. There has been a dramatic improvement in the quality of life for these young children and the arm is none the worse since collateral channels developed rapidly (although this could not have been known beforehand and thus the experimental procedure would have been difficult to justify in advance). This procedure coupled with later correction of Fallot's tetralogy has meant that the outlook for many of these children is now near normal.

Catheter balloon septostomy

Another spectacular success was Rashkind's invention of the technique of catheter balloon septostomy in which a hole is created between the atria in children with transposition of the great arteries; before his invention children with transposition always died young because the right and left circulations were entirely separate; septostomy permitted mixing of blood in the atria and hence survival. The technique was the first time that cardiac catheterisation became a treatment as opposed to a diagnostic procedure.

Palliative and corrective procedures

The principle of trying new medical procedures is surely right. Some, like those described above, will gain acceptance and others may not but without trying them progress will be slow. All these procedures may be classified into those that are palliative, which improve a child's health without necessarily touching the underlying condition, and those that are corrective, which restore normal anatomy. The word 'cure' is not appropriate here. Even after an apparently simple corrective procedure the heart will remain abnormal; for example the tiny scar resulting from stitching an atrial septal defect may be sufficient to trigger abnormal rhythms and hence palpitation in later life.

Eisenmenger syndrome

In some forms of congenital heart disease the sufferer looks blue. This discoloration (called cyanosis) is due to the right heart blood (which lacks oxygen) crossing a defect in the 'wrong' direction. The blue blood appears in the left heart and is thence carried to the body where it can be seen most easily in the blue discoloration of the lips. In order for this right to left shunting to take place there has to be both a defect, which is commonly in the ventricular septum, and something that stops blood flow into the lungs either as pulmonary stenosis or as a result of high resistance in the pulmonary arteries. The latter condition is known as the Eisenmenger syndrome, after the man who described it. Minor increases in pulmonary artery pressure are inevitable with the passage of the years in children with left to right shunts. But some have such a severe increase that the pressure equals or exceeds the blood pressure in the rest of the body whereupon blood starts flowing in the reverse direction and cyanosis develops. Any pronounced increase in pulmonary artery pressure is alarming because it prohibits successful surgery for cardiac defects (the defect can actually be closed successfully but subsequently the right heart fails and the patient dies). Fear of an abnormal rise in pulmonary artery pressure is an additional reason for recommending early surgery to correct serious left to right shunts.

Outlook for those with Eisenmenger syndrome

Once the Eisenmenger syndrome has developed patients may live reasonable lives for many years but the blood gradually becomes thicker as more and more red cells are produced by the body.

Increasing fatigue may be improved by taking off blood but stroke is a real risk and pregnancy is literally fatal both for mother and child. Fortunately women with cyanotic heart disease rarely become pregnant but when they do termination is advisable. People with the Eisenmenger syndrome usually die in middle life and death is generally sudden. The only surgical option is heart-lung transplantation which can bring about an improvement in the quality of life but since experience with the procedure is very limited we do not know whether the victim lives longer.

What causes congenital malformations?

The cause of congenital malformations is largely obscure, with one exception. German measles (rubella) in a mother during the first few months of pregnancy can produce a characteristic pattern of malformations including those of the heart. No other infection acquired during pregnancy has been clearly shown to have such an effect, although suspicion is sometimes cast on virus infections that produce a high fever. Certain drugs, for example warfarin, can predispose to congenital malformations. Some malformations tend to run in families but often we are not sure how they are inherited. No doubt the basic fault lies in the genetic make up of the unborn child but at the moment we know of no way of identifying or manipulating the genetic codes. But advances in gene technology may change this and present us with a new set of moral decisions. Already antenatal diagnosis of some malformations is possible by echocardiography but the information comes too late for that pregnancy to be terminated and heart surgery for the unborn child is not practicable yet. The future for these infants with heart disease is extraordinarily difficult to foresee.

9 Related circulatory disorders

High blood pressure

High blood pressure (hypertension) has already been discussed as a risk factor for coronary heart disease in Chapter 4 but it is important in its own right. Blood pressure is like all human characteristics in that there is no 'normal' level. It varies from person to person and from moment to moment. People with persistently high levels are more likely, however, to suffer from arterial damage which may lead to a heart attack or stroke. The damage to the arteries develops over decades and then takes the form not only of atheroma but also of bulges or 'blow-outs' (aneurysm) and other disorders of the arterial wall.

How common is it?

In any population the range of blood pressure is like the range of heights; most people have a measurement that falls round the middle of the range with a few very high and a few very low. The few at the top, who are the ones at risk from arterial disease, do not differ materially from their neighbours with slightly lower pressures; like tall people they are at the extreme end of a range rather than suffering from some specific disorder such as pneumonia with a single identifiable cause. When doctors are faced with such a harmful biological variant they like to give it a label, and in this case the term 'essential hypertension' is sometimes heard. Very rarely high blood pressure does have a cause such as coarctation of the aorta (Chapter 7), or an excess production of the hormone adrenaline, or a narrowing of an artery to a kidney. In these rare situations correction of the underlying fault may return the pressure to normal.

Are there any symptoms?

High blood pressure is totally silent — you cannot tell when your

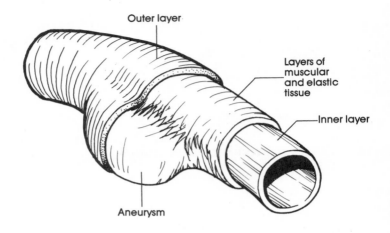

Outer layer

Layers of muscular and elastic tissue

Inner layer

Aneurysm

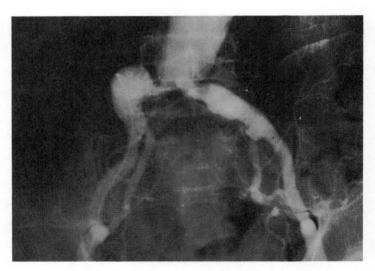

An arterial aneurysm is a swelling of one part of the wall of an artery which has been weakened. This may grow until it bursts due to the pressure of blood flow through it.

blood pressure is high. But the damaging effects of high blood pressure can be detected during a medical examination since the heart shows signs of strain, protein leaks out of the kidney into the urine, and the small arteries in the back of the eye (retina) become irregular and tortuous. These changes, however, are the result of longstanding high blood pressure and treatment should really begin earlier. Hence the value of screening. We all tend to put our blood pressure up when frightened so many measurements may be necessary before treatment is advised.

Weight, salt, and exercise

People with high blood pressure are often overweight, so diet is therefore the first line of treatment. A reduced salt intake may also lower blood pressure and exercise is beneficial. We do not know why this is, but it may be connected with salt loss through sweating. Claims have been made that high blood pressure can be lowered by yoga and other relaxation techniques but there is no convincing proof of this.

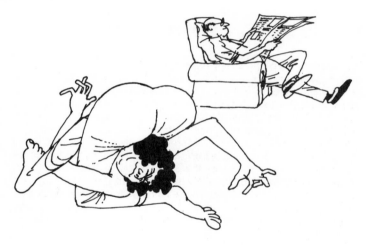

Drug treatment

The mainstay of treatment for high blood pressure is drug treatment. There are four main categories:
- *Diuretics or water pills*: act by eliminating salt and water;
- *Beta blockers*: reduce the nervous drive to the heart and circulation;
- *Vasodilators*: relax the muscular tone in the walls of the arteries and veins, these include the *angiotensin converting enzyme (ACE) inhibitors*;
- *Calcium antagonists*: probably also act to reduce the muscular tone in the arterial wall.

Drug treatment is often life-long

These four categories of drugs differ in the way they work and are often used together. Treatment generally starts with one, then rather than give a larger dose which may increase the possibility of side effects, another drug is added, and another if necessary. Once started, treatment should generally be continued for life or until the risks exceed the benefits. These modern drugs are very safe and very well tolerated but they may cause an undue fall in blood pressure and therefore a tendency to lightheadedness or faintness on getting up quickly, particularly after a bath, or exercise, or in a hot stuffy room where you are drinking alcohol (all circumstances in which the blood pressure can plummet). This complication is more likely in the elderly and may be a reason for stopping treatment in this group.

Stroke

Stroke is caused by an interruption of the blood supply to the brain, generally from a blocked or burst artery. For many people a stroke is truly a fate worse than death — one side of their body is paralysed, vision on that side is lost and, if the dominant side of the brain is involved (left in a right-handed person) the ability to speak is affected. This classic effect of a stroke has many variants. For example in some victims speech alone is affected. Several small strokes may leave the victim unable to swallow or to control his bladder, and demented, or the stroke may be slight and very temporary causing no more than a few minutes clouding of a segment of the field of vision. The terms ischaemia and infarction are used for the brain (cerebrum) as well as the heart, so you may hear about cerebral infarct, transient ischaemic attack, or cerebrovascular accident (CVA).

What causes a stroke?

The cause of a stroke usually lies in the arteries to the brain, which have been damaged by high blood pressure. Occasionally, however, the fault lies in the heart. Small blood clots which develop in the left ventricle or atrium can travel in the blood stream to lodge in one of the arteries of the brain. Clots have a regrettable habit of travelling that way because such a large proportion of the output of the heart goes to the brain. But these clots can end up anywhere, in a leg for example. Experience has shown that these clots are most likely to develop in patients with mechanical heart valves,

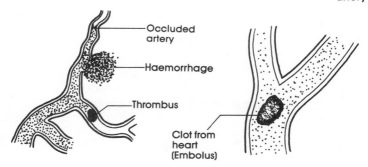

How strokes happen.

those with rheumatic mitral valve disease, and less commonly in those with big, 'baggy' hearts caused by cardiomyopathy or extensive myocardial infarction. The first two groups must receive anticoagulant treatment with warfarin if they are to avoid clot formation and the third group probably should.

Prevention is vital

Treatment of an established stroke is so unsatisfactory that prevention, whenever possible, is vital. Once a part of the brain is damaged it never recovers. Careful retraining can permit some recovery of function but motivation is usually the key factor here. You should remember that people who have had a stroke often retain understanding even though they cannot communicate. They can usually hear and see and interpret what is going on around, but cannot express themselves; all too often the grotesque attempts at speech emerge as meaningless grunts. Women, who live longer than men, often linger on after a stroke no doubt envying their menfolk who died suddenly from a heart attack.

Aortic aneurysm

A bulge or 'blow-out' of the aorta, an aortic aneurysm has disastrous consequences. High blood pressure is yet again a culprit, but a basic weakness of the wall of the aorta is another incriminating factor, seen, for example, in those who have a widespread weakness of the connecting tissue of the body (called Marfan's syndrome). Any part of the aorta may be affected. In the abdomen, a gradual blow-out leads to widening of the aorta, which is then prone to leak blood once the diameter of the aneurysm exceeds 5cm. This can be identified by ultrasound examination and the aneurysm should be removed surgically.

Problems in the thoracic aorta

In the chest (thorax) some widening of the aorta is commonplace as we get older. Slowly developing aneurysms are seen from time to time but here a peculiar catastrophe is dissection of the thoracic aorta. In this condition a tear occurs in the inner lining of the aortic wall. Blood under high pressure tracks along the wall between the inner and outer layers and separates them; rupture of the outer wall leads to sudden death from internal bleeding. Other possibilities are tearing of the aortic valve or coronary arteries or leakage of blood into the pericardial sac as the dissection tracks back to the heart. If the victim survives, urgent surgical repair to replace the torn segment with a tube of Dacron can be life-saving. Once again though, prevention through early control of high blood pressure is the better medicine.

Lung disease

The heart and lungs are closely related and normally these relations are friendly. The right heart pushes blood through the lungs to pick up oxygen and get rid of the waste carbon dioxide. The left heart receives blood from the lungs and drives it round the body. When the relationship is strained, the fault may rest with the heart, as we have seen when failure of the left heart leads to congestion of the lungs and shortness of breath, but it may rest in the lungs.

Cor pulmonale

Many diseases of the lung, such as chronic bronchitis, emphysema, and lung fibrosis, cause loss of lung tissue, including the network of arteries and veins that carry the blood. This in turn increases the resistance to blood flow through the lungs, raises the pressure in the pulmonary artery, and eventually leads to right heart failure. This sequence of events is called cor pulmonale.

Embolism

A minor function of the small arteries of the lung is to act as filters. Particles in the blood, which might block the arteries to the brain etc are thereby prevented from entering the left heart and causing a stroke or heart attack. The only common particle to be found in the veins is a clot. We probably form small clots in our veins quite frequently but normally dissolve them as soon as they form. When our clotting mechanisms are working overtime, for example after an operation or when we are confined to bed, approximately one third of us develop a clot (or thrombus) in the deep veins of the leg. This deep venous thrombosis impedes the drainage of blood from the leg which therefore becomes swollen, hot, and painful. Bits of the clot can break off and move with the blood to lodge in the lungs. This is known as pulmonary embolism. If the migrant clot (or embolus) is small it goes undetected. A somewhat larger clot blocks off a part of the blood supply to the lungs which subsequently becomes an infarct causing pain in the chest and shortness of breath. A very large clot blocks off the entire blood supply to the lungs and is another cause of sudden death.

Anticoagulant drugs

Several small clots developing one after the other may gradually block off the blood supply to the lungs and cause a relentless increase in pulmonary artery pressure which leads to progressive right heart failure. All these conditions must be treated with anticoagulant drugs. A very large pulmonary embolism may be treated with streptokinase or surgery.

Primary pulmonary hypertension

Primary pulmonary hypertension mimics lots of small pulmonary emboli. The word primary, like the word essential, implies that the cause is unknown and like essential hypertension in the rest of the body the fault seems to lie in the small arteries that become progressively narrowed as the arterial wall thickens with scar tissue. The disease usually affects young women and is generally well advanced before it is diagnosed because the early stages are symptomless. Mild shortness of breath and tiredness are the initial complaints but these often progress so that effort may also cause a feeling of faintness. The diagnosis may be suspected on physical examination but usually has to be confirmed by cardiac catheterisation. Unfortunately, treatment is unsatisfactory, although vasodilators may help and anticoagulants seem to improve life expectancy. Occasionally heart-lung transplantation may be indicated for these patients.

Pericardial disease

The fibrous sac around the heart, the pericardium, seems to have little use in normal healthy people. When the pericardium becomes inflamed, the condition is known as pericarditis. This is not uncommon and is usually caused by a virus infection. Someone with pericarditis generally feels unwell with a fever and muscular aches and pains, and pericarditis is suspected when cardiac-like pain develops with these symptoms. The pain has subtle differences, for example deep breaths hurt and the pain tends to be eased by sitting up and leaning forward. The doctor can sometimes hear a pericardial rub — a characteristic scratchy sound above the normal heart sounds — and the electrocardiogram may confirm the diagnosis. Pericarditis also occurs in other situations, for example after a myocardial infarct, when the pericardium overlying the dead heart muscle becomes inflamed. Typically, the patient seems to be getting over his heart attack but continues to experience grumbling chest pain which worries everyone until the rub is heard, whereupon there is great relief that the pain does not mean continuing ischaemia. Rarely patients suffer relapses of pericarditis of unknown cause and some pericarditis is inevitable after heart surgery but again rapidly resolves. The outlook is excellent. Treatment with aspirin in full dosage (up to two tablets every four hours) is helpful.

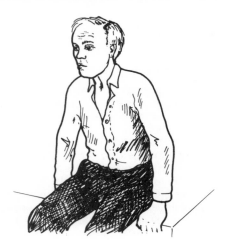

The pain of pericarditis tends to be eased by sitting up and leaning forwards.

Constrictive pericarditis

Constrictive pericarditis is a special longstanding type of pericarditis in which the pericardium becomes converted into hard scar tissue which constricts the heart. Logically this condition might be expected after an attack of viral pericarditis but this has never been proved and patients with constrictive pericarditis seldom remember having had pericardial pain. The cause is therefore unknown with one exception — tuberculosis can inflame the pericardium and cause constriction. People with constrictive pericarditis have the symptoms of right heart failure. Once the diagnosis is suspected and confirmed by echocardiography, the treatment is surgical — to remove the pericardium. The results are very successful.

Tumours

The pericardium may be affected by tumours which grow into the fibrous sac and when severe can compress the heart and stop the flow of blood through it. This is known as cardiac tamponade and is in effect a sudden severe form of pericardial constriction. Cancer of the lung, breast, and Hodgkin's disease are the commoner causes but the same picture may also be seen after excess radiotherapy to that part of the chest. The diagnosis may, yet again, be established by echocardiography. Unfortunately treatment is very unsatisfactory.

Haemopericardium

Finally, the pericardium may fill with blood (haemopericardium) and compress the heart. The causes of this condition include aortic dissection, cardiac rupture after a heart attack or accidental damage, and bleeding from a tumour or after heart surgery. Urgent surgical treatment is essential for haemopericardium.

Miscellaneous disorders

The heart may suffer damage from knife wounds and in accidents, for example when the chest is impaled on the steering wheel of a car. Damage of this nature is known as trauma and is probably more common than we suspect. Sometimes the victim of a major road traffic accident will have his broken bones and cuts treated and then a few days later he starts to deteriorate, whereupon the damage to his heart is noticed. Treatment is obviously surgical in the first instance to control bleeding, but becomes medical if complications such as arrhythmias or heart failure arise.

Heart tumours

Tumours of the heart are incredibly rare. The most common variety is a fatty growth (myxoma) which usually develops in the left atrium and causes trouble either by obstructing the flow of blood, causing faints and heart failure, or by throwing off clots, which cause stroke, etc. Occasionally tumours from elsewhere migrate to the heart. The diagnosis of a cardiac tumour can be established by echocardiography and, when appropriate, the tumour should be removed.

Glandular disorders

Some glandular disorders affect the heart, but for practical purposes the only important one is overactivity of the thyroid gland (hyperthyroidism or thyrotoxicosis). This causes the heart to beat faster and may therefore be the explanation for palpitation. Atrial fibrillation and heart failure may occur if the overactivity goes untreated. Once suspected, however, the diagnosis is easily established by blood tests and treatment is very satisfactory. This disorder, like constrictive pericarditis, left atrial myxoma, and several others that affect the heart, is not common but together these conditions cause much suffering. Since all can be effectively treated once diagnosed, there is a powerful argument for having a heart specialist in every district hospital.

Cardiac 'non-diseases'

Finally, there is a group of cardiac 'non-diseases'. Over the years terms such as 'soldiers heart', 'athletes heart', 'neurocirculatory asthenia', and 'hyperventilation' have all been used to describe disorders in which the victim complains of symptoms which suggest heart disease, such as palpitation and shortness of breath. Although slight evidence of a cardiac abnormality may be found in these people, the heart is in fact normal. Unfortunately, this may be very difficult to prove and only the uneventful passage of many years establishes the diagnosis with certainty. After enjoying a decade or more of ill health and the opinions of numerous specialists, someone with a 'non-disease' may have the possibility of heart disease so firmly ingrained in their mind that he or she will reject any suggestion that their heart might be normal. In these people a cardiac neurosis is firmly established and treatment is generally unrewarding, although they often derive great comfort from alternative or complementary medicine.

10 Rhythm disturbances (arrhythmias)

If your heart is beating with an abnormal rhythm you will feel this as palpitation. Most of us experience palpitation occasionally as a strong, regular, thumping sensation in the chest after exertion or emotion. But an arrhythmia feels different and can be extraordinarily difficult to describe. The commonest type of arrhythmia is called an extrasystole and this is usually felt as a missed heart beat.

Extrasystole

An extrasystole is a single, abnormal beat that interrupts the usual rhythm of the heart. It occurs when the heart would normally be relaxing (during diastole) and is followed by a relatively long pause. You are not usually aware of the extrasystole itself because the heart is only half filled and the beat is small. But the subsequent pause creates an alarming sensation, almost as if your heart were going to stop. Then the next beat comes with a great thump because the volume of blood it has to pump is larger than normal.

We all have them

Sooner or later everyone experiences extrasystoles. They are frightening on the first occasion, may recur several times a day especially before going to sleep at night, and often go away for some weeks only to reappear later without rhyme or reason. Extrasystoles are sometimes made worse by stimulants such as coffee. Very occasionally they indicate heart disease and for this reason you should consult your doctor. Once any underlying heart disease has been excluded, however, you can be reassured, and no further action is required. If the extrasystoles are very frequent or distressing, treatment with drugs may be necessary, but the results are not very satisfactory.

Tachycardias

An extrasystole is a single abnormal beat: a run of extrasystoles is called a tachycardia. There are different types of tachycardia depending on which part of the heart is causing the problem. Supraventricular tachycardia originates in the atria or atrioventricular node. It is usually caused by a short circuit. The fault was probably present at birth but the tachycardia does not become apparent until adult life. This is perhaps because children cannot describe what is happening to them, they just do not feel right. The usual symptom is a fast, regular heartbeat that starts suddenly, lasts minutes or hours, and then stops with equal suddenness. You may feel faint, especially when it begins, but usually the attacks are not too troublesome. Like extrasystoles, attacks of supraventricular tachycardia generally occur unpredictably.

Coping with supraventricular tachycardia

Various physical manoeuvres will stop an attack once it has begun. The most successful is to lie down, take a deep breath, and then breathe out against a closed throat. (This is rather like 'pushing' during childbirth or when opening your bowels.) The tachycardia will often stop as you let the breath go. Drugs are helpful if the attacks are very frequent, but because they take some time to work they are not really useful in preventing single, isolated attacks. We sorely need a drug in an aerosol that can be inhaled into the lungs to reach the heart within seconds. The outlook for people with episodes of supraventricular tachycardia is excellent as the attacks seem to disappear in later life.

Ventricular tachycardia

Ventricular tachycardia feels rather similar to supraventricular tachycardia but originates in the ventricle. It is experienced by people with established heart disease, usually coronary heart disease. The outlook for people with this problem is not good and drug treatment is almost always necessary.

Atrial fibrillation

The normal rhythmic, electrical activity of the atria may break down and this is known as atrial fibrillation. In this condition electrical miniwaves course around the atrial muscle in a chaotic fashion. Coordinated muscle contraction stops and the ventricles are bombarded with electrical impulses. The function of the atria, to act as a boost pump for the ventricles, is thereby lost and in someone with cardiac damage this may cause heart failure. More often, however, the heart tolerates atrial fibrillation quite well but the sufferer feels distinctly uncomfortable. Atrial fibrillation may occur from time to time (paroxysmal) or it may become continuous.

Symptoms and treatment

The symptoms are attacks of palpitation in which the heartbeat (actually the ventricular beat) is totally irregular and with no pattern as there is for example with a series of extrasystoles. The heart rate may be fast if the sufferer also has some other form of heart disease such as hyperthyroidism or coronary or rheumatic heart disease. If, however, the fibrillation occurs by itself without other evidence of heart disease (termed lone atrial fibrillation) the heart rate may be almost normal. Treatment of paroxysmal atrial fibrillation aims to prevent the attacks with drugs like quinidine. Treatment of established atrial fibrillation is directed at controlling the rate of the heartbeat with digoxin.

Ventricular fibrillation

Ventricular fibrillation is, of course, a totally different type of arrhythmia in which the chaotic ventricular rhythm means that the heart stops pumping blood and that the victim dies.

Slow rhythms

Hitherto we have been concerned with extra beats and fast rhythms but at the other end of the scale are the various forms of slow rhythm. You may be aware of your heart slowing down or pausing but more usually you will feel faint or actually faint (syncope). Some young people faint when they see something unpleasant, for example blood. This is because the vagus nerve, which is normally responsible for slowing the heart rate at rest, stimulates the heart too much. These fainters usually lose the tendency as they mature but as we age further the reflexes that control our circulation become less efficient so that we sometimes feel faint or light-headed when we get up quickly. This has a different cause, namely a brief drop in blood pressure as we change posture. In younger people the blood pressure, and hence the blood supply to the brain, is maintained because the muscular tone in the arteries and veins in the lower part of the body increases suddenly when we stand. Blood is shifted back into the central circulation from the pool in the legs and pelvis. Unfortunately older people lose this reflex. The condition is called postural hypotension and is particularly likely to occur in hot conditions when the blood vessels are relaxed, for example after a bath or sitting in front of a hot fire; after alcohol; or when taking certain drugs, particularly those used to treat high blood presure. Unfortunately, postural hypotension can lead to accidents and falls.

Stokes-Adams attacks

Pauses in the rhythm of the heart will lead to unconsciousness after a few seconds. This may be caused by either a faulty electrical connection between the atria and ventricles (called heart block) or a fault in the origin of the electrical impulses (sinus arrest). The victim may not survive his first attack but he generally does, regaining consciousness in less than a minute. These faints have a characteristic pattern which was first recognised by two Irish physicians (Stokes and Adams) and whose names are sometimes used to describe the attacks. Other features, in addition to the abrupt loss and recovery of consciousness, are the deathly white appearance of the victim during an attack, the absence of a pulse, and the flushing which occurs during recovery.

Diagnosing the rhythm disturbances

These disturbances of cardiac rhythm occur unpredictably and are seldom witnessed by doctors — we only rarely see what happens during an attack of palpitation or a faint. The diagnosis has to be made from what the patient and his family tell us and what a physical examination and electrocardiography show, and from techniques such as ambulatory electrocardiography (see Chapter 2).

Treatment

For some people with extrasystoles and frequent tachycardias, treatment with drugs may be required. Occasionally surgery to remove an abnormal electrical pathway may be helpful. For patients with Stokes–Adams attacks a cardiac pacemaker is essential.

Cardiac pacemakers

Cardiac pacemakers are yet another example of the way in which technology has transformed the lives of people with heart disease. The simplest cardiac pacemakers are matchbox-sixed cans comprising a power source (usually two lithium-iodine batteries), an electrical circuit, and a plug which takes a lead to the heart. The system is implanted by a cardiologist, who inserts the electrode into a vein, generally one just behind the collar bone, positions the tip in the right ventricle, and attaches the other end to the pacemaker unit which is then inserted under the skin of the chest wall. The procedure is performed under a local anaesthetic and takes about 45 minutes.

How does it work?

The electrical circuitry, which is often a minute chip, senses the normal activity of the heart and, provided your heart is beating at a reasonable speed, just sits there quietly. If, however, your heart pauses or goes unduly slowly then the pacemaker cuts in and prevents a blackout. The heart is stimulated from an unusual site, from the right ventricle, and the beat may feel different to you but it is perfectly adequate for daily living. If your heart beat is permanently slowed then the paced rhythm permits an almost normal lifestyle. The usual standby rate of the pacemaker is 70 beats per minute.

Long lasting and effective

Modern pacemaker batteries last many years and at the end of that time the pacemaker can be changed quite easily under local anaesthetic. People who have Stokes–Adams attacks are often elderly but physically youthful with a heart that works well apart from the electrical fault. Indeed there is a strong suspicion that the less hardy do not survive their first blackout, so that pacemaker centres see only a selected population of youthful old people. Pacemaker treatment is extremely effective. You no longer need to be terrified of the next unprovoked blackout and can resume a normal life, including driving. The complications of treatment are rare, but the electrode may become dislodged in the early

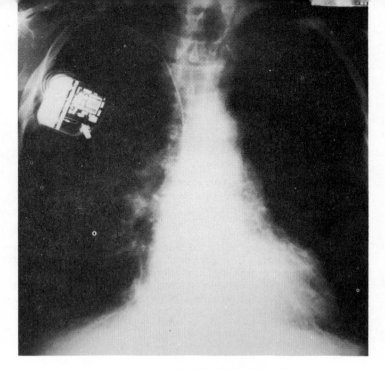

X-ray of a permanently implanted heart pacemaker.

days, the system may become infected in which case it has to be removed, and rarely the pacemaker may erode through the skin.

Sophisticated technology

Modern pacemakers are even more sophisticated than the one I have described. There are dual chamber systems that can pick up the electrical signals from the atria and transmit them to the ventricles. But two leads are necessary, the units are bigger, and the additional expense is seldom justified.

Programmable pacemakers. Programmable pacemakers contain a small metal switch which can be activated by a magnet incorporated into a 'programmer' positioned over the unit on your skin. This allows the doctor to change the standby rate of the pacemaker or the voltage output. About 15% of the pacemakers used in Britain are programmable. Their main advantage is that they allow doctors to programme the units after implantation in such a way that battery life can be conserved.

Rate responsive pacemakers. Rate responsive pacemakers are able to increase their rate of discharge in response to the needs of the body, for example by sensing the rate of breathing. The best known of these devices detects bodily movement. Any activity such as walking is sensed by a crystal incorporated in the pacemaker which then increases its rate of firing. The only problem with this type is that you may have an episode of tachycardia whenever you travel by British Rail (don't we all?) but for some people this is a small price to pay for an improved ability to exercise.

Automatic, implantable defibrillators

The latest developments in pacemaker technology have introduced systems for patients with disabling attacks of paroxysmal tachycardia — a critically-timed, electrical impulse can stop an attack. There is also an automatic, implantable defibrillator that can sense ventricular fibrillation and deliver a current of sufficient intensity to restore regular rhythm. This can be used when all else fails. Several hundred of these have been implanted in patients in North America.

Simplest is often best

All these more sophisticated electrical devices are expensive and complicated, which in practice means that they are more likely to go wrong. Since pacemaker failure may mean discomfort and death, there is great merit in sticking to the simpler systems in all but desperate cases. At 1989 prices these cost around £500 to £600, whereas the more sophisticated systems are several times more expensive.

Living with a pacemaker

One month after you have had a cardiac pacemaker implanted you can lead a normal life, including driving. Because pacemakers can sense high frequency electrical signals, however, it is possible that some types of electrical apparatus may stop them working properly. This is certainly a theoretical risk but in practice there is seldom a problem. The reported incidence of pacemaker interference is very low indeed. There were five possible occurrences reported out of the many thousand pacemaker users in Britain in a two year period. Furthermore, instead of actually being inhibited by outside electrical interference, all modern pacemakers will begin pacing the heart at a fixed, fast rate so that you know something is wrong and can move away from the source

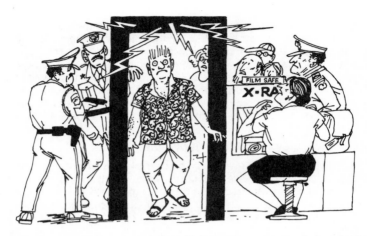

of the trouble. Domestic appliances and all the pieces of electrical apparatus that we come into contact with in normal daily life will only interfere with a cardiac pacemaker if they are faulty. Don't be too alarmed by the sort of warning notice seen, for example, on microwave ovens.

Creating your own interference

Using the large muscle on the front of the upper chest, which is responsible for arm movement (pectoralis major), is occasionally a cause of electrical interference. Thus pacemaker patients may occasionally feel palpitations while shaving or doing things that involve contraction of this muscle. If this complication is particularly troublesome, the cure is to reposition the pacemaker.

A security problem?

The metal parts of cardiac pacemakers, for example the titanium can, are picked up by detectors at airports and some large department stores. Remember therefore that you may be accused of carrying an explosive device as you attempt to board an aircraft or of shoplifting by a store detective! For these and other reasons, you should always carry the card that is given to you by the pacemaker centre at the time of implantation.

11 Working and living with heart disease

Work

People with heart disease are not allowed to do certain jobs. The chief reason for this is the risk of sudden incapacity through a cardiac arrhythmia, particularly ventricular fibrillation which causes sudden death. The risk of such a catastrophe is very small but even the more common and less serious rhythm disturbances which cause lightheadedness or an uncomfortable sensation in the chest are frightening and distracting. Likewise cardiac pain can lead to loss of concentration. Therefore anyone liable to experience these conditions may not undertake jobs in which a temporary loss of concentration could have serious consquences.

Which jobs can't you do?

No-one with important heart disease may be an:
- Airline pilot;
- Merchant seaman;
- Driver of a mainline railway engine;
- Heavy goods vehicle or public service vehicle driver;
- Or indeed hold any job in which his or her sudden ill health could result in harm to others.

Unfortunately, despite legislation and guidelines, disasters still happen, for example a coach driver suddenly loses consciousness at the wheel and his passengers are killed and injured.

Some risk is inevitable

Complete freedom from risk cannot be ensured. One in 10 people with coronary heart disease drop dead as their first sign of heart trouble and to try and guard against this eventuality would involve going to ridiculous lengths. All employees in responsible jobs would have to be screened and those who might be liable to develop heart disease would have to be weeded out. From the

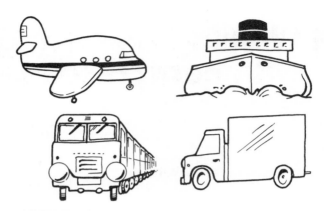

Forbidden accupations.

heart specialist's viewpoint a workforce of young women would be highly desirable — on the other hand, older men do have a few useful qualities! While this illustration is facetious it does have a serious intent in that it introduces the concept of relative risk.

Relative risk

The risk of sudden incapacity through cardiac arrhythmia is greatest in those with the most extensive heart disease. Working men with no evidence of heart or circulatory disorders have a very low risk of heart attack, around 1 per 100 men each year. For those who already have some evidence of cardiovascular disease, for example angina pectoris or a previous heart attack, then the risk is 12 times greater. People with good cardiac function and a single unimportant coronary arterial narrowing have a trivial risk and are going to enjoy good health for many years, whereas those with poor cardiac function, extensive coronary narrowing, and recent heart attack are much more likely to have ventricular fibrillation. The risk can be measured and costed. A level of acceptable risk can be agreed by employers and advisory bodies such as British Rail, the Civil Aviation Authority, and the Department of Transport. In fact this already happens for the organisations mentioned and private employers can and should do likewise. The concept of relative risk is sensible and fair and most employees will readily cooperate with such a policy.

Fear is a problem

The whole subject of work and heart disease is bedevilled by the fear of sudden incapacity and death. This fear makes employers reluctant to re-employ men with heart disease. A fatal recurrence while at work would be bad for the corporate image! This fear may be the stimulus to health screening as the employer can then be shown to have done his best, although as we have already seen, the benefit to the employee is doubtful.

Promoting better health

Employers would actually do better to spend their money on promoting measures to encourage the primary prevention of coronary heart disease.
- Smoking should be banned in offices and on the shop floor. A smoking room may be set aside for addicts.
- The canteen should offer healthy foods with plenty of vegetables and fruit.
- Facilities for physical recreation should be provided.

Some enlightened companies already do all this to their immense credit and to the longer term health of their employees. Inevitably though, some men will develop heart trouble, usually a heart attack; then what should the policy be?

Work seldom harms

If the psychological or physical pressures of work could be clearly shown to cause heart disease then a policy of not re-employing men with heart disease would be justifiable. But the truth of the matter is that work seldom did anyone harm, whatever old wives say. Men do get promoted beyond their natural level of ability, do experience psychological pressure, and fail to cope. The subsequent heart attack may perhaps be advanced by such stress but it would probably have happened anyway. Interestingly, heart attacks do often happen when relief, in the form of retirement, has just arrived. Physical work is more likely to protect against a heart attack than promote one.

Retirement

The experience of a heart attack concentrates the mind wonderfully. Many people take stock of life and decide to retire but they should be aware that to do so on grounds of ill health may not be financially advantageous. And for some retirement can be a boring prelude to senility and death. Retirement from work is not usually necessary for most patients with heart disease. They differ from people with arthritis, for example, whose mobility is restricted by stiff, painful, joints. Very rarely in patients with heart disease does shortness of breath or fatigue limit the ability to work but when this is truly the case retirement is necessary.

Outlook after heart attack

Most victims of a heart attack will recover and will seem normal to the casual acquaintance. Predicting the future for anyone is always impossible but doctors can at least place such a person in a category according to the chance of a future attack. Granted the individual's permission, medical advice can then be given to the employer. Most employees should return to their former jobs. A few should be advised to retire because their external appearance belies the extensive cardiac damage. Paradoxically the psychological pressures of work may no longer bother the individual, they have become relatively unimportant. Those in physical work should increase their duties gradually.

Valve replacement and bypass surgery

Similar advice applies to people who have had heart valve replacement or coronary bypass surgery. These operations are generally undertaken nowadays before the heart muscle has become damaged and a good recovery is to be expected. As with someone who has had a heart attack, you may actually feel and perform better afterwards because you have changed your attitude to life. Return to full time work at three months after heart surgery is usual. The reason for not returning to work is generally that the employer is fearful of further absences through sickness and takes this opportunity to offer the job to a younger man.

If the heart muscle is damaged

The above comments apply to those whose hearts work adequately. As described in Chapter 7, however, damaged heart muscle, whatever the underlying cause, will deteriorate further when subjected to physical work. Anyone therefore who has had heart failure should be advised to retire from physically demanding work and the same should probably apply to those whose left ventricle is not working well, especially if it deteriorates on exercise (see Chapter 2).

Driving

Advice about driving and heart disease is set out in a booklet entitled *Medical Aspects of Fitness to Drive* which is available to all doctors. The advice is based on the distilled wisdom of a panel of heart specialists who meet regularly with the medical branch of the Department of Transport. While not infallible, the advice represents a responsible compromise between infringing personal liberty and protecting other road users from the consequences of a heart attack at the wheel. There is an important distinction between the ordinary driving licence and a vocational licence because the consequences of an accident resulting from ill health are so much more serious for the vocational driver.

Regulations for vocational drivers

The regulations that apply to vocational or professional drivers are very strict. Vocational in this context means holders of heavy goods vehicle or public service vehicle licences together with some others, but not including minicab drivers. No-one with significant heart disease may hold a vocational licence, because of the risk of sudden incapacity through ventricular fibrillation. The word significant conceals a small loophole through which some drivers can pass. The risk of ventricular fibrillation in coronary heart disease is in fact minute in those with good cardiac function and localised coronary disease.

After a small heart attack some drivers can regain their licence providing they:

● Survive in good health for one year;

● Satisfy a heart specialist that they are truly in good health;

● Pass certain tests which include electrocardiography, stress testing, and coronary arteriography.

The regulations after bypass surgery are similar.

After other forms of heart surgery the chances of regaining a vocational licence are even smaller and anyone who has to take anticoagulants (blood thinning treatment) cannot hold a vocational licence. This therefore debars anyone with a mechanical heart valve. No-one with a pacemaker or persisting cardiac arrhythmia can hold a vocational licence. In general, young people with heart problems who are thinking about a job as a vocational driver should be discouraged.

Ordinary driving licences

The motor car is one of life's essential ingredients. The regulations concerning heart disease and ordinary driving licences recognise this and only prohibit driving for approximately one month after heart surgery, pacemaker implantation, or heart attack, and permanently for any patient with unexplained and untreated blackouts or near blackouts.

Insurance

Anyone with continuing health problems that might affect their ability to drive *must* inform their insurance company and the medical branch of the Department of Transport. If in doubt consult your doctor.

Living

To offer advice about life is both presumptuous and difficult — it all depends upon you and the risks you wish to take. A book of this nature can only attempt to spell out some of the options, starting with advice about that major scourge — coronary heart disease.

The bon viveur *v* the killjoy

Health educators have persuaded governments that coronary heart disease is a terrible burden to the community and that vigorous effort is needed to stamp it out. Many heart specialists, however, are conspicuous by their silence on this issue. We are conscious that stamping out premature coronary heart disease is desirable but realise that worse fates can lie in store for the elderly who do not die suddenly from a heart attack. Moreover life is to be enjoyed not endured. At one end of life's spectrum lies the overweight bon-viveur who drops dead, cigarette in hand, at a

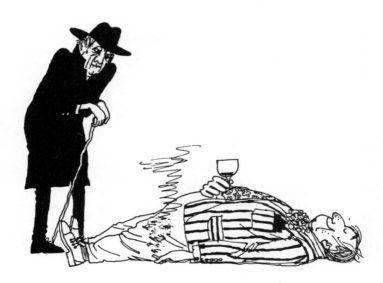

party; it may spoil the party but what does he care? At the other end lies the killjoy who has eschewed life's pleasures but survived to a ripe old age; at least he can take pleasure in saying 'I told you so'.

It's your life

Life has to be a compromise. Smoking must be stamped out because the burden to the overall health budget is too great. Beyond that dictat the public and individuals may receive advice but they should feel free to choose their own destiny. Some may wish to jog and have an extra two years or so of life; others might prefer to watch television and forgo the possible extra time. Some will want to keep dairy farmers in business; others will wish to patronise the health food shops. Health screening clinics should be avoided since they bring misery and little benefit beyond the blood pressure check. And a little alcohol may lubricate the machinery of life.

A suspended sentence

When heart disease does strike, a death sentence is imposed. The only real change, however, is that you have been forced to think about your life span, while the rest of us can continue to ignore our fate. There is really no excuse nowadays for anyone to be ignorant of the risk factors for heart disease, but if this was so then firm counselling should take place once heart disease is diagnosed. Otherwise day to day living may continue unchanged for most. Only when the heart is severely damaged does it become necessary to make alterations to the home or lifestyle. Angina can be controlled, survival in good health after a heart attack is the norm, and all that is required is sensible planning for the future, taking into account the results of risk stratification (see Chapter 4) and the opinion of the heart specialist.

Exercise

In general exercise is good for the heart but does not have to be compulsory. A gradual increase in physical activity after the onset of coronary heart disease is beneficial. The type and level of activity does not matter much but it should be enjoyable. Nor should coronary heart disease affect normal sexual activity, which is said to be equivalent to walking up two flights of stairs. Of course no two couples are the same but then neither are any two flights of stairs. If physical activity brings on chest discomfort or shortness of breath then you should see your doctor.

91

What about lifting?

For some reason patients with coronary heart disease are advised to avoid lifting. Probably the advice is received at the bar rather than the health centre but the belief that lifting may strain the heart is held by many people. The effort of lifting does involve a surge in blood pressure with little change in heart rate as opposed to dynamic exercise such as running or cycling or swimming in which the heart rate increases with little change in blood pressure. The cost to the heart in terms of an increased need for oxygen and other nutrients is greater for the former but the heart can cope perfectly well provided, as always, that the effort is increased gradually. Confusion may arise because unaccustomed or inexpert lifting of heavy weights strains the muscles of the chest wall and causes pain which may be misinterpreted as cardiac pain.

Damaged heart muscle

These suggestions do not apply to people whose heart muscle is damaged. As outlined in Chapter 7, the damaged heart has limited resources and effort should therefore be kept to a minimum. This applies regardless of the cause of the cardiac damage. Firm guidelines cannot be laid down since everyone is different. But to take an extreme case, the patient with progressive, severe heart failure. He might be advised to

- Move his bed and washing facilities downstairs;
- Only go outside when the weather is fine and still;
- Avoid washing up, gardening, and housework;
- Sleep and rest in a chair and avoid excitement.

The outlook for someone who is so ill is so poor, however, that alterations to the home which involve spending money are seldom justified. Similarly, moving to a better environment, for example to get away from hills or the British winter, may end in disappointment with the victim dying and a spouse left in an unfamiliar and friendless place.

Bypass or heart valve surgery

After coronary bypass or heart valve surgery a return to normal life is usual. For children and young people with heart disease individual counselling is necessary. Generalisations are unwise but certain careers are not open to them, including those mentioned earlier in this chapter and the Services. Sometimes physical effort has to be minimised in an attempt to conserve cardiac function, for example in someone with congenital aortic stenosis. Striking a balance between growing up normally and minimising physical effort is extraordinarily difficult but a reasonable compromise is to permit normal play but prevent competitive sports.

Modern treatment means a better quality life

Advice about lifestyle used to be a prominent feature of books about heart disease. This is no longer so. One reason is that medicine used to have little else to offer patients with heart disease, so attention to posture, sleep patterns, and such assumed undue importance. Another reason is that our understanding of the effects of heart disease is now much greater, so that there are fewer unknowns to frighten us. The most important reason, however, is that advances in treatment and especially progress in medical technology have been so enormous that virtually everyone with heart disease can enjoy a better quality of life. Having said that it is important to remember that no one can be cured.

Index